Understanding Allergies

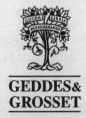

GEDDES & GROSSET

ISBN 1 85534 327 4

Printed and bound in the UK

2 4 6 8 10 9 7 5 3 1

Contents

Contents

Contents

Introduction

Human beings have developed a complex system to defend themselves from the millions of potentially harmful organisms and agents that might invade the body at any time. These invaders include bacteria, viruses, parasites, microscopic moulds and fungi, and a range of chemical toxins. As will be described in the following chapter, the system that has developed to counteract these, the immune system, is extremely complex and has developed a diverse range of mechanisms to oppose and eject invaders from the body. An equally complex control mechanism has developed along with this so that the immune system reacts only when necessary and for the length of time appropriate to ensure that the invader poses no threat. The complex physiological mechanisms involved are not yet fully understood.

The main features of the immune system are that it can adapt, it is specific, and it can remember and recognise 'self', i.e. it does not act against its own tissues.

With such a complex and intricate system, it is not surprising that, on occasion, various parts do not operate as they should. This may be for a variety of reasons. It may be because some of the mechanisms are missing or not working properly in certain individuals or the control functions of the system may be deficient in some way. There are a number of reasons why these defects can occur.

This book examines some of the ways in which the immune system goes wrong and the conditions that result from this. It also looks at the role of the immune system in transplant surgery.

In some people the immune system can be acting perhaps too well, and this is called being hypersensitive. This inappropriate action of the immune system is the cause of allergies such as asthma and hay fever. The immune system overreacts to substances that in most people cause no harm and many different symptoms result, according to which part of the body is affected. Instead of protecting the body, this particular type of immune response causes damage and in some cases can lead to death. As far as is known, allergies provide no useful function.

One important characteristic of the immune system is its ability to distinguish between 'self' and 'non-self'. A normally functioning immune system can recognise its own tissues and does not react against them. Sometimes this ability is lost and the immune system begins reacting with its own body cells, causing severe damage to various organs and tissues. This 'action against self' gives rise to conditions known as autoimmune diseases, which are probably the result of a fault in the control mechanism of the immune system. Autoimmune diseases include some types of diabetes and thyroid disorders and various haemolytic anaemias. Rheumatoid arthritis is another condition that is believed to be the result of an autoimmune response.

In some individuals, certain parts of the immune system do not work properly or are missing altogether; for example, some people cannot produce certain types of white blood cells that are crucial in fighting disease. Conditions arising from this type of problem are known as immunodeficient diseases. These conditions may range from mild and treatable ones to very serious ones, which do not lend themselves to treatment and can often be fatal. Such deficiencies in the immune system can either be congenital or arise as a result of certain adverse conditions, including disease, malnutrition or use of toxic drugs, e.g. those used in the treatment of cancer. The most well-known example is Aids (Acquired Immune Deficiency Syndrome). In this case, a virus seriously impairs the immune system, leaving the patient unable to fight off infections. Death from lung infections or cancer usually follows.

The function of the immune system is to protect the body from 'foreign' and 'invading' agents. While this is essential for human survival, it presents a problem in the case of transplants. An immune system that is functioning normally will recognise the transplant organ as foreign and will try to destroy it, resulting in its rejection. In the early days of transplant surgery, this was the single most important reason for failure. Nowadays, immunosuppressive drugs that reduce the normal immune response are increasingly successful in stopping the transplanted organ from being rejected. However, this reduced immunity then leaves the patient prone to other types of infection.

Hence it can be seen that the immune system plays a vital role in maintaining health and life. Any malfunction or breakdown in the system can lead to a wide range of conditions, some of them fatal. A great deal remains to be discovered about the immune system, and one major area of research is its role in the development of cancer. It is known that cancer patients have an increased rate of infection, and immunological abnormalities have been identified in some of those affected. At the same time, cancer is more common than would be expected in patients with immunodeficiencies and in those on immunosuppressive drugs. The fact that the immune system has a role in the development of cancer is accepted, but the mystery of its precise role remains to be unravelled. Recently it has been found that one type of cell in the immune system, known as natural killer T-cell, attacks tumour cells or those infected with a virus and is therefore vitally important. Manipulation of the components of the immune response that activate these killer cells may provide the key to the development of anti-cancer drugs in the future.

1

The Immune System

The human body is continually exposed to a range of disease-causing agents, including bacteria, viruses and parasites. In order to protect itself from such potentially dangerous agents, the body has developed a system – the immune system – which can recognise foreign substances within the body and eliminate them. In addition to the micro-organisms that the body encounters every day, the immune system also recognises as '*foreign*' cancer cells and transplanted organs, e.g. heart, kidney and skin grafts. A properly functioning immune system therefore presents problems of rejection for transplant patients. (*See* Chapter 13).

In some people, the immune system is defective and provides fewer defences against infection than it should. This is known as *immunodeficiency* and may be the result of several factors, including malnutrition, infection and old age.

In other individuals, the immune system is hypersensitive. It overreacts to certain harmless substances that would not bring about the same reaction in people with a normally functioning immune system. This inappropriate reaction, which instead of protecting the body against disease is itself a cause of disease, is known as an *allergy*.

Components of the immune system

Any agent recognised as foreign by the immune system is called an *antigen*. The body encounters a vast array of antigens, numbering in the thousands, and the immune system has therefore had to develop a complex system in order to enable it to react appropriately.

Immunity consists of a non-specific element and a specific element. Non-specific immunity is inborn, usually present from birth, and reacts in the same way to all antigens. This type of immunity is mediated by particular cells that ingest and digest invading micro-organisms. In contrast, specific or acquired immunity is learned and is a consequence of an encounter with a specific antigen. Specific immunity also has the ability to 'remember' previous encounters with the same antigen and adapt its response.

The immune system is largely composed of three different kinds of cell and three kinds of protein, all with a specific function to perform in the body's response. All six components are found circulating in the blood in some form or other.

Cellular components
The cellular components are:

- *Granulocytes* – these are the most numerous nucleus-containing cells in the blood. They can engulf antigens entering the body and, using potent enzymes within the granulocyte, can digest the invader, rendering it harmless.

- *Monocytes* – these comprise only a small percentage of the cells in the bloodstream. When found outside the blood system they undergo changes in structure and are called macrophages. Like granulocytes, macrophages can engulf and digest foreign substances. In addition, monocytes alter the antigens in a way that makes the immune response of the third kind of immune system cell, the lymphocyte, more effective.

- *Lymphocytes* – in some respects these are regarded as the most important cells in the immune system. They are present in very large numbers in the body, in excess of a million million. There are two main kinds: T lymphocytes and B lymphocytes (also referred to as T cells and B cells). T lymphocytes outnumber B lymphocytes by 5:1.

Both T lymphocytes and B lymphocytes are remarkable in that they will react with only one particular molecular shape, in much the same way as a lock works with only one key. Each lymphocyte will 'lock' into only one particular antigen. Lymphocytes are capable of responding to millions of foreign antigens but not to the body's own proteins.

B lymphocytes and their direct descendants are responsible for the production of immunoglobulins or antibodies. When a B lymphocyte recognises an antigen it begins to divide rapidly. The activated daughter cells of this division make enormous amounts of antibody, which are released into the blood, the tissue fluids and body secretions.

T lymphocytes are responsible for what is known as cellular immunity. Like B lymphocytes, they can recognise antigens and become stimulated but instead of producing antibodies their daughter cells attack and kill antigens directly. They also have the ability to kill cells that have become infected with micro-organisms such as viruses. T lymphocytes can additionally kill abnormal and 'foreign' cells, and are implicated in the rejection of organ transplants and may be important in some forms of cancer. Finally, T lymphocytes also have the ability to increase or suppress the immune response by regulating other components of the system.

Both T lymphocytes and B lymphocytes have the ability to 'remember' previous exposure to a specific antigen, so enabling more effective destruction of this foreign substance on future exposure.

Proteins

The three kinds of proteins in the immune system are the cytokines, complement proteins and immunoglobulins (also called antibodies). All three are found in blood serum (the liquid part of blood).

- *Cytokines* – these are largely responsible for regulating the immune response. They may be secreted by lymphocytes or monocytes, in which case they are known as lymphokines and monokines respectively. The cytokines may act in several different ways to regulate the immune response. They may increase an ongoing immune response, others may instruct cells to proliferate and some may act to suppress the ongoing response. This ensures that the immune system is active when appropriate but not overactive, so preventing damage to the body.

• *Complement proteins* – these are a group of non-specific proteins that act along with immunoglobulins and one another to develop an effective immune response. Complement proteins bind to the antibody-antigen complex, which aids the ingestion and digestion of the antigen by the immune system cells. These complexes are also important in local histamine release.

• *Immunoglobulins* – there are thousands of different kinds of immunoglobulins or antibodies. Each different type of antibody has developed in response to a specific antigen and helps in its removal from the body. Although antibodies cannot penetrate living cells, they are present throughout the body and on its surface. Antibodies work in a variety of different ways: some react with toxic chemicals to inactivate them; others coat the surface of micro-organisms to aid their removal by phagocytes; yet others prevent viruses from entering cells; and another group is able

15

to kill bacteria directly. Antibodies can be divided into five main categories:

Immunoglobulin G (IgG) – the most abundant antibody, comprising about 75 per cent of the total immunoglobulin level in the blood. It is active in response to bacteria, viruses and toxins. It is the only antibody that can pass across the placenta from mother to foetus, giving the baby some initial protection against infection. IgG is also a 'blocker' that is capable of preventing another antibody, IgE, from triggering an allergic response.

Immunoglobulin A (IgA) – this is present only in small amounts and is found in body secretions such as tears, sweat, saliva and breast milk. The presence of IgA in breast milk means that temporary immunity can pass from mother to baby. High concentrations of IgA are found in colostrum, suggesting that it may have a particular protective effect in the gut of the newborn. IgA is mainly concerned with protection at the mucosal surfaces of the lungs and digestive system.

Immunoglobulin M (IgM) – this is the largest immunoglobulin and is the first to appear in the immune response. In combination with complement IgM, it can kill bacteria directly.

Immunoglobulin D (IgD) – the least understood of the immunoglobulins. It is present only in small quantities and is thought to be important in the development of certain kinds of white blood cells.

Immunoglobulin E (IgE) – the antibody that is central to the development of allergic diseases. High levels are found in many people with allergies. It is found primarily in the mucous surfaces of the respiratory system and gut. It may also have a beneficial role in defence against parasites.

The immune response

The cellular components of the immune system, including the lymphocytes, which are responsible for the production of antibodies, are produced in the bone marrow. From here they are released into the bloodstream and can then migrate and meander through the body tissues. Millions of these scavenger white blood cells and lymphocytes are found in body tissues. In the normal course of events, these cells eventually enter the lymph system and from there return to the bloodstream to repeat the cycle. (Figure 1.1).

At any one time, there are enormous numbers of white blood cells continually 'patrolling' the body tissues on the lookout for 'foreign' material (antigens). When an antigen enters the body, on the surface of, say, a bacterium, one of these lymphocytes recognises the antigen and initiates the immune response.

The lymphocytes respond by dividing and forming many activated daughter cells. The daughter cells of the B lymphocytes produce huge quantities of specific antibody to the particular antigen. These are released into

Figure 1.1: Activation of a mast cell

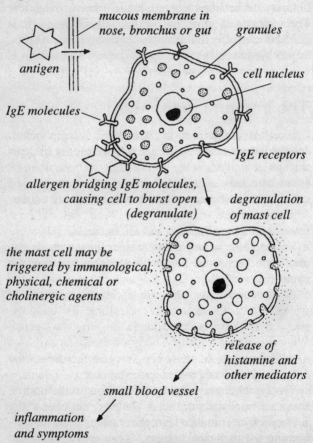

mucous membrane in nose, bronchus or gut

granules

antigen

cell nucleus

IgE molecules

IgE receptors

allergen bridging IgE molecules, causing cell to burst open (degranulate)

degranulation of mast cell

the mast cell may be triggered by immunological, physical, chemical or cholinergic agents

release of histamine and other mediators

small blood vessel

inflammation and symptoms

the circulation, tissue fluids and body secretions, and bind to the antigens that stimulated their production. The antibody binding has several consequences that eliminate or help eliminate the foreign material. Firstly, the antibody clumps antigen together, which makes it easier to remove. Antibody also greatly increases the rate at which white blood cells can ingest antigen. It can also kill foreign matter directly, and finally can coat and neutralise poisonous substances.

The daughter cells of the stimulated T lymphocytes do not make antibodies but get rid of antigens in other ways:

- they attack and kill bacteria directly
- they kill cells that have become infected with certain germs like viruses
- they kill some abnormal and foreign cells

The combined response of the immune systems, including the action of T lymphocytes together with the production of antibodies by B lymphocytes, leads to the death of invading microbes.

The allergic response

An allergic reaction is a particular type of immune reaction that, instead of protecting the body, causes damage by producing unnecessary symptoms. As in the normal immune response described above, recognition of a particular antigen stimulates lymphocytes to divide rapidly, forming cells that make antibody against that substance.

The antibody then binds onto the antigen. However, in the case of allergy, the capacity to differentiate between potentially harmful substances from harmless ones is absent. In an allergic response the antigen is called an *allergen*.

Allergic reactions are always directed against substances that are harmless in themselves, unlike the more usual immune response, which is directed against harmful, disease-causing agents. In allergy, it is the allergic response itself that is harmful. In non-allergic people, for example, dust mites, pollen grains and shellfish cause no health problems at all, but in allergic individuals these can cause severe symptoms, illness and in some cases death.

There are two phases in the development of an allergic reaction. The first is the initial setting up or *sensitisation* of the allergic response, which leaves a person allergic to a particular substance. The second phase is the triggering that leads to an attack when the person meets the same allergen again. The first encounter with the allergen does not provoke a reaction, but if an individual becomes sensitised, each subsequent encounter provokes an allergic response.

In the 1960s, two British immunologists, P. G. H. Gell and R. R. A. Coombs, published a classification of hypersensitive or allergic reactions. Despite certain limitations, this classification remains the most satisfactory and is still widely used. Under this scheme, allergic reactions are classified into four different types. However, many people prefer to use the word 'allergy' to refer only to the immediate Type I hypersensitivity.

The four types of reaction are:

- **Type I** reactions are immediate or anaphylactic reactions in which allergens combine with specific IgE antibodies and there is a subsequent release of powerful chemicals from mast and other body cells. Disorders included in this group are the well-known allergic conditions of hay fever, asthma and eczema.
- **Type II** reactions occur when antibodies react with antigens in cells or tissues or when antibodies on the cell surface make them more likely to be destroyed by monocytes. Included in this type are many autoimmune diseases and blood transfusion reactions where there is a mismatch of blood types.
- **Type III** reactions involve immune complex reactions resulting from antigen-antibody complexes being deposited in body tissues or blood vessels. Disorders in this group include serum sickness, farmer's lung and possibly rheumatoid arthritis and other autoimmune diseases that are described in Chapter 11.
- **Type IV** reactions include delayed sensitivity reactions and are caused by sensitised T lymphocytes after contact with a specific antigen. This is a cell-mediated response and antibodies are not involved. This delayed type of reaction is involved in contact dermatitis, some forms of drug sensitivity and transplant rejection. In contact dermatitis, the allergens are called

haptens, typical examples being hormones and other drugs. The haptens combine with proteins in the skin to form a complete allergen. (See *contact dermatitis* in Chapter 5)

Type I allergic reactions

Even before a particular allergen is encountered for the first time, a small number of B lymphocytes have the precise molecular structure which is able to 'lock into' that type of substance. In the initial encounter, a lymphocyte is stimulated to divide rapidly, and its daughter cells produce large quantities of IgE antibodies to the allergen. Symptoms do not arise on this occasion because the number of cells involved is small. However, this *sensitisation* or *primary response* primes the lymphocytes to recognise the allergen in subsequent meetings and enables it to be dealt with more ferociously. Later encounters with the same allergen result in symptoms that vary in severity according to the individual.

Mast cells

In the allergic response, another type of cell, the mast cell, has been found to play an important role, particularly in respiratory allergies such as hay fever. The mast cells are found concentrated in the linings of the nose, sinuses, lower respiratory tract and the skin. The surface of the mast cells is full of specialised receptor sites to which the antibody IgE is attracted. It is estimated that there are about 300,000 such sites on each mast cell. Each mast cell contains tiny 'packets' of chemical granules, each surrounded by its own membrane. When an allergen combines with the IgE antibody attached to a mast cell, changes in the cell membrane result. This in turn triggers the release of chemicals known as mediators from the granules inside the cell, a process known as *degranulation*.

It is these mediator chemicals, released from the mast cells, that bring about the symptoms associated with allergic reactions, most notably allergic inflammation. One of the earliest mediators to be identified was histamine. Other more powerful, longer-acting chemicals were also known to be present, but it was not until the 1980s that the nature of these was made clear. It was found that the cell membranes of the mast cells and other tissue cells nearby release arachidonic acids, which in turn lead to the production of more powerful compounds such as leukotrienes and prostaglandins. Leukotrienes are known to be thousands of times more powerful than histamine and have a longer-lasting effect. There are 20 different types of prostaglandins, with a variety of effects in the body. Prostaglandins are involved in regulating the immune response, particularly in inflammation. The prostaglandins produced in the aftermath of a mast cell reaction are responsible for keeping up the attack on an invader.

The combination of the chemicals released by the

mast cells is responsible for producing the three reactions manifested in allergic reactions:

- dilation of small blood vessels with increased permeability (or leakiness) – the basis for urticaria, angioedema, nasal blockage and allergic headache.
- smooth muscle spasm, which produces the contraction of the airways typical of asthma, and is also probably responsible for the spasms that accompany gastro-intestinal allergy.
- increased secretions, which are evident in allergic conjunctivitis, ear disorders, asthma and hay fever.

It is known, for instance, that all three chemicals are active in asthma.

Histamine contracts the central bronchial passages while leukotrienes are mainly responsible for the narrowing of peripheral airways. Prostaglandins, a group of fatty acids, also constrict the air passages.

Reaction to histamine produces the thin watery mucus and provokes the itching and sneezing typical of hay fever.

Fluid leaking from small blood vessels is responsible for the typical weals of urticaria and the swelling of the deeper layers of the skin and underlying tissue that occurs in angioedema. (*See* Chapter 6). White blood cells called eosinophils congregate at the site of an allergic reaction. Like mast cells, eosinophils contain powerful chemicals within granules. When released these can cause destruction and death of tissue.

The presence of eosinophils is common in many allergic conditions, and they are also present in people with worm infestations. Their presence in both these gives a clue, in evolutionary terms, as to why mast cells may be present in the body, even although they appear to serve no useful function but, on the contrary, seem to act against a person's best interest.

Parasitic worms in the body stimulate the production of IgE, which causes mast cells in the vicinity of the worms to degranulate. Among the substances released from the granules is a factor that strongly attracts eosinophils to the worms. The eosinophils attack the worms and also attract antibodies to them, which help their destruction. The worms become coated with mucous and are washed away through the gut. The IgE/mast cell system is well suited to help clear the surface of the digestive system, the lung, the nose and the skin of worms and other parasites. The inflammatory response produces symptoms such as coughing, scratching, sneezing, running nose and diarrhoea, all of which helps clear these surfaces of the parasites. In some parts of the world where worm infestations are still common, this 'allergic-type' reaction may be important. In the more developed parts of the world such parasitic infections are less frequent and can be treated with drugs. However, the mast cells still remain and cause allergic reactions to a whole range of harmless substances.

2

Allergies

Allergies were first described by Hippocrates in the 5th century BC, although it was not until the beginning of the 20th century that the term 'allergy' was first used. Hippocrates recognised asthma and recorded the spasmodic nature of the illness. He suggested that the cold precipitated the condition. Hippocrates also recognised allergies to food and observed that while cheese was an excellent food for most people, in some people even the smallest piece caused a severe reaction. The terms 'eczema' and 'asthma' were both in use around that time.

Since then many allergies have been described, although the cause of them was often not known. John Bostock, a physician in London, was the first person to describe the clinical symptoms of hay fever in a paper to the Royal Medical Chirurgical Society in the early 19th century. However, it was not until 1872 that Charles Blackley would demonstrate that pollen was the cause of hay fever, one of the most common allergies.

The word 'allergy' was first used by an Austrian paediatrician, Clemens von Pirquet, in 1906. He used it to describe an altered capacity to react, i.e. the abnormal reaction some people have to common substances. At that time children were immunised against diphtheria using an antitoxin. Von Pirquet noticed that a few children became violently ill after these injections and some of them died. He suggested that the first injection of antitoxin had brought about an altered reactive state in these children and used the word 'allergy' to describe it.

In 1921, two German scientists, Prausnitz and Kustner, carried out an experiment that demonstrated that allergy was caused by something in the blood serum. However, it was not until 1967 that two Japanese doctors, a husband and wife team called Ishizaka working in the United States, identified the factor involved as the antibody immunoglobulin E (IgE). In the same year, Voorhorst identified the house dust mite as an important cause of allergy.

What causes allergies?

An allergy is an adverse reaction to a substance that causes no problem at all in most people. Any substance that causes such a reaction is known as an 'allergen'. The most common allergens include substances such as pollen, moulds and foods. It is specific proteins in these substances that act as the allergenic agent. To provoke an allergic reaction, these proteins must be soluble in water so that they can dissolve in the watery secretions of mucous membranes of the nose, lungs and digestive tract. The proteins must also be small enough to pass through these protective membranes and gain entry into the body, and yet be big enough so that when they encounter cells of the immune system, they can trigger an allergic reaction. Some allergens that are too small to provoke an allergic reaction by themselves combine with other proteins in the body to trigger a response. For a protein to act as an allergen it must be relatively common in the environment. Adverse reactions to an allergen do not occur until the allergen is encountered for at least the second time. On initial exposure, the body becomes sensitised to the specific allergen and produces an allergic reaction on subsequent encounters. However, not all proteins that satisfy these criteria act as allergens. It is not known why some proteins act as allergens and others do not.

Some allergens are encountered only intermittently; for example, many foods that cause allergies may be eaten only occasionally. Other allergens are seasonal in nature, most notably pollens which cause hay fever in susceptible individuals. Pollens from a wide variety of plants can cause hay fever, and so at least some of them are around for a good part of the year. Fortunately for hay-fever sufferers, many of them are susceptible to only one or two types of pollen and so their period of suffering is limited to particular pollination periods. Other types of allergen are present all year round, for example the house dust mite, which is implicated in respiratory allergies, so there is no period of relief for sufferers.

The symptoms caused depend on how the allergen comes into contact with or enters the body. On this basis allergens can be divided into inhaled allergens, contact allergens, ingested allergens and injected allergens. Examples of these different types of allergen can be found in Table 2.1.

Some allergies such as hay fever are very common, and it is estimated that as many as one in ten people suffers from this condition. Others are very rare, particularly some of those caused by exposure to certain chemicals at work. The abundance of a particular allergen in the environment influences how many people are affected by a particular allergy.

Are allergies on the increase?

The number and range of allergies are often said to be increasing. One estimate suggests the numbers of victims are increasing by about 5 per cent a year. Indeed, some people seem to be allergic to modern-day living and are allergic to many substances in their environment. It is estimated that at least 40 per cent of the UK population will have an allergic reaction at some time in their lives. So many children now have asthma that the government recently issued guidelines regarding the use of inhalers in schools.

Although some of this increase in the number of people suffering from allergies is probably because of better diagnosis and understanding of allergy, a proportion

Table 2.1: Types of allergens	
Inhaled	Pollen – various tree, weed, grass and flower pollens Dusts – house, flour and grain, dust from hay Animal dander and hair Fungal spores Chemicals – industrial, household, insecticides Insect debris – mites in flour and grain
Contact	Plants Clothing Drugs when applied as ointments or creams Cleaning agents such as soap, shampoos, detergents Cosmetics, e.g. deodorants, perfumes, hair dyes Metals, particularly nickel and chromium Chemicals – inks, dyes, oils
Ingested	Foods, particularly wheat, milk, eggs, nuts, shellfish Additives in food
Injected	Drugs Insect stings, e.g. wasps, bees, hornets

will be the result of a real increase in the number of people suffering from allergic conditions. Several explanations have been put forward to account for this increase.

One explanation for the increased number of food allergies reported is that children are being exposed to a greater number of foodstuffs at a younger age. They can therefore become sensitised to a range of foods before their own immune system is fully developed. The increase in the number of people allergic to nuts, particularly peanuts, is thought to be the result of early exposure to this food. Delaying exposure of infants to foods such as wheat and eggs is advised in an attempt to reduce symptoms and possible development of allergies related to these foodstuffs. (*See* Chapter 7). It has also been suggested that the vast number of additives used in foodstuffs, some 3500, may also contribute to the increasing number of food allergies, although there is little evidence to support this as yet. The average person now swallows 4.5 kilograms of food additives every year – about ten times more than thirty years ago.

Exposure to a wide range of chemicals, including artificial ones, in the environment is also thought to play a part in the increase in the number of people developing allergies. There is increasing evidence that the rising incidence of asthma is a result of the higher levels of air pollution, particularly in cities. This pollution comes from two main sources: traffic exhausts and industrial emissions. There is some evidence that nitrogen dioxide from car exhausts and the ozone produced by the action of sunlight on them together act to damage the lining of the lungs. The surface of the air passages in normal, healthy lungs is lined with ciliated cells (cells with small hair-like protuberances). These cells waft particles and mucus in the lungs back up the air tubes and keep the surface of the lungs clean. Nitrogen oxides, even in quite low concentrations, interfere with the action of the ciliated cells so that they do not work so efficiently. Any airborne allergens, such as pollen grains, that enter the lungs are therefore less likely to be wafted out. They will be in contact with the lining of the lung for a longer period and so are more likely to provoke an allergic response. In this way, pollutants may not act as allergens themselves but create the conditions to promote attack.

The presence of very low concentrations of ozone and pollen together in the atmosphere may cause asthmatic attacks, although the presence of either one of these in low concentrations is unlikely to do so alone. It appears that the two factors act together to cause an allergic response.

The whooping cough vaccine has recently been implicated in the increase in the atopic allergies of eczema, asthma and hay fever. A study based at the Churchill Hospital in Oxford involving 2000 patients born between 1975 and 1984 found that children vaccinated against whooping cough are 50 per cent more likely to develop eczema, hay fever and asthma later in life. The same study also found that being given broad-spectrum antibiotics as a baby puts children at a three times greater risk of developing allergic disease. A history of allergy in the mother was additionally found to be an important factor. It is believed that the administration of the whooping-cough vaccine provokes an abnormally strong immune response to allergens, while broad-spectrum antibiotics, which kill a wide range of bacteria, may disturb the development of the immune system in the infant.

Another study investigating the relationship between the whooping-cough vaccine and asthma found that the rate of asthma was five times higher amongst those children who were immunised than those who were not. Hoyet another study, however, showed the opposite effect, with children who were not vaccinated more likely to develop wheezing.

The reasons for the increase in cases of allergic conditions are not clear. There may well be several factors involved, which interact with each other. The benefits of whooping-cough vaccine still outweigh the possible negative effects, but more selective administration of vaccines and antibiotics should be considered.

Why do some people develop allergies and others do not?

The tendency to develop allergies often runs in families and so there is obviously a genetic component involved in some cases. Families who develop allergies are referred to as *atopic*. In these families there is a strong tendency for several, if not all, the family members to suffer from one or all of the following allergies: asthma, hay fever (*allergic rhinitis*) and eczema (*atopic dermatitis*). The tendency to develop these conditions is more commonly inherited from the mother than the father. Recent scientific advances in determining the genetic link in allergy have pinpointed two of the genes responsible for asthma, although several others are also likely to be involved. It is probably only a matter of time before other genes responsible for various allergies are discovered.

Although genetic inheritance is important in determining who will develop allergies and who will not, it is not the only factor involved. Allergic parents do not always have allergic children, and vice versa. Environmental factors also play an important role. Firstly, individuals have to be exposed to the allergen to develop an allergy to it. Secondly, the timing of the first exposure may be important. Many children often develop allergies as babies before their immune system is well developed but grow out of them as they get older.

There are probably a number of other factors that are important in determining who develops allergies. Further studies of allergy, the role of the immune system and the genetic component will undoubtedly reveal more answers to this complex question.

3

Respiratory Allergies

Seasonal and perennial rhinitis – hay fever

The nose and the eyes are the parts of the body most frequently affected by allergy. Hay fever, or more properly *seasonal rhinitis*, is perhaps the most common and the one with which most people are familiar. It affects the upper respiratory tract, the eyes and nose. It is estimated that about one in ten people suffers from the disorder.

Allergic rhinitis simply means inflammation of the nose caused by an allergen. Seasonal rhinitis is usually caused by pollen grains in the air and occurrence peaks from late spring to early summer in Europe and Australia. Perennial rhinitis occurs all year round, with varying severity, and is usually caused by house dust or animals.

The nose has a moist, corrugated lining and is designed to filter out particles in the air that we breathe to prevent them from reaching the lungs. It is not surprising then that the nose is a primary site for allergies. Pollen grains, spores and dust are all caught up in its lining and can stimulate an allergic reaction.

The onset of hay fever usually occurs in childhood and early adolescence, and is more common in boys. The symptoms vary in severity from one individual to another, and some children grow out of the condition while others carry it on into adulthood.

Seasonal rhinitis

Seasonal rhinitis (hay fever) is the commonest form of allergic rhinitis and is caused mainly by wind-borne pollen released into the air by trees and grasses. It can also be caused by airborne moulds.

Hay fever, a term coined in the 1830s, is misleading. Hay fever has nothing to do with hay and rarely produces fever in the sufferer. It was Charles Harrison Blackley, in 1872, who first showed that the symptoms of hay fever were the result of a seasonal allergy caused by exposure to pollen grains.

Pollen grains contain the male sexual cells of plants, which fertilise egg cells to produce seed. They are transferred from one plant to another by the wind or on the bodies of insects. For the hay fever sufferer, wind-borne pollen causes the greatest threat. Pollen grains are produced and released into the atmosphere in huge numbers. It is the widely distributed plants that are also allergenic that are the most important cause of hay fever.

There are three groups of plants the pollen of which is a major cause of allergy:

- grasses
- trees
- weeds

In addition, pollen from cereals and certain flowers, e.g. chrysanthemums, can also cause hay fever.

In Europe and Australia, grass pollens are the most common cause. In Britain, hay fever caused by grass pollen occurs from mid-May to early August and peaks in June and early July. The exact time at which the pollen arrives depends on the weather that season; if the spring weather is colder than usual, pollen release may be delayed. There is also a geographical variation in the 'hay fever season' for a given species. For example, it will occur earlier in southern Europe than in the north of Scotland where the climate is cooler.

In Britain, tree pollination begins as early as February or March with the alder and elm, followed by the oak in June. Pollen from all these trees is implicated in hay fever allergy whereas that from chestnut and beech trees is rarely involved. Other trees are important causes of hay fever in different countries, e.g. the birch in Sweden and the olive in southern Europe.

In the United States, the pollen of ragweed is the commonest cause. Ragweed pollinates between August and October so hay fever there is most likely to occur in the autumn.

The cultivation of oil seed rape (*Brassicus napus*) has been increasing in Britain over the last few years and may also be implicated in hay fever.

The amount of pollen being carried in the atmosphere is very dependent on weather conditions. On dry, sunny, windy days the concentration of pollen in the air is at its highest. On such days, pollen can be carried great distances on warm air currents, sometimes far into the atmosphere. As the air temperature cools in the evening, the pollen can fall back in concentrated clouds to lower levels. Rain and windless conditions reduce the concentration of pollen grains in the air.

Weather forecasts in many countries now include a pollen count. This is expressed as the number of pollen grains per cubic metre of air during a 24-hour period. A count of over 50 is likely to cause symptoms in many hay-fever sufferers. However, later on, even lower counts can be troublesome as a sufferer becomes more sensitive as the season progresses.

Symptoms of seasonal rhinitis

The symptoms of seasonal rhinitis are very similar to those of the common cold with which it can be easily confused. Initially, the nose, the roof of the mouth, the throat and the eyes begin to itch, either gradually or abruptly. This is accompanied or followed by the three main manifestations – sneezing, watery discharge and blocked nose.

Sneezing is caused by the irritation of the nasal lining and bouts of 5–20 sneezes can occur. This is often the first sign of an attack. Sneezing and itching result from the effects of histamine released in the nose during the allergic reaction to pollen.

Histamine release in the nose also causes the secretion of watery fluid. The sufferer is subject to a constantly running nose that necessitates continual sniffing and blowing. The running nose will continue as long as the sufferer is exposed to the pollen.

The third main symptom in hay fever, a blocked nose, is the result of the swelling of the nasal membranes. This is not helped by nose blowing, unlike the case with a cold, and if the nose is completely blocked, sniffing to clear the watery discharge is prevented. In short, the runny yet blocked nose together with bouts of sneezing can make life miserable.

In severe cases, headaches, irritability, depression, loss of appetite and insomnia can also occur. The length and severity of an attack depends on the length and amount of exposure to the allergen and can vary from a short sneezing bout to several days.

Other symptoms

The eye can also be affected by hay fever. The eye itself is unique in that most of it cannot mount an allergic response. However, the surrounding tissues can. The conjunctiva, the membrane that covers the white of the eye and lines the inside of the eyelid, is involved in allergic reactions. During an episode of hay fever, the conjunctiva may become inflamed and the blood supply to it increases, making it swell. The eye looks red and inflamed. Itching encourages rubbing of the eye, which only makes the itching and swelling worse. In severe cases, swelling can close the eye and it can be painful to look at bright lights. Tears are secreted in an attempt to wash away the allergen, resulting in watering eyes.

Diagnosis

The seasonal nature of the symptoms of hay fever make the diagnosis relatively easy in most cases. Timing of the onset of attacks can also help identify the precise pollen responsible, although patients are rarely sensitive to only one kind.

Diagnosis of seasonal rhinitis is also supported by physical symptoms and confirmation of the presence of eosinophils and mast cells in the nasal secretions – the white blood cells active in allergic responses. These cells are present in 80 per cent of hay-fever suffers. Skin tests may be useful to confirm or identify the pollens responsible.

Treatment

Antihistamines
Antihistamines are particularly useful in relieving the symptoms of runny nose, sneezing and watering, itching eyes, but they do not help in the relief of blocked nasal passages.

Antihistamines have been used in the treatment of

hay fever for over 50 years. Although they are successful in relieving symptoms some of these drugs, such as
Piriton or Fabahistin, have a sedative effect and users of
them often become drowsy. Normal working is difficult,
and those taking them are advised not to drive, operate
machinery or take alcohol. However, in the early 1980s
a new generation of drugs was introduced in which this
side effect was much reduced or absent altogether.
These newer antihistamines, such as terfanadine (brand
name Triludan), astemizole (Hismanal), loratadine
(Clarityn) and cetrizine (Zirtek), have been widely used
to treat the symptoms. Some of them could be bought
over the counter, but there is now some concern over
three particular types: terfanadine, astemizole and loratadine. Heart problems such as irregular beats have been
observed in a few people on these drugs, and so they are
now available only on prescription.

Triludan acts very rapidly and symptoms are usually
relieved within a few hours of taking the drug. It does
not stay in the body for long and so doses have to be tak-
en two or three times a day. Hismanal does not have
such an immediate response but has the advantage of remaining in the body for longer and needs to be taken
only once a day. Neither should be taken during pregnancy as they can have deleterious effects on the foetus.

Decongestants

These are used to clear nasal blockages associated with
hay fever. They act by shrinking the size of the blood

vessels in the lining of the nose and so reduce swelling. They are usually taken in the form of nose drops and are popular because they can bring instant relief. However, the relief is short-lived and repeated doses are required. In the case of earlier drugs used as decongestants, over-use often resulted in worse congestion. They also became less effective the more they were used. More recently developed compounds, such as oxymetazoline and xylometazoline, are more powerful, longer-lasting and have fewer side effects. It is still recommended that they should not be taken for more than two or three weeks at a time.

Taken in the form of tablets, decongestants can raise blood pressure. Patients with a tendency to high blood pressure should not use them without periodic monitoring by their doctor. Care also has to be exercised if the patient is on any other form of medication. Consultation with a doctor is advised in these cases.

Decongestants are additionally often found combined with antihistamine preparations.

Antiallergic drugs

These act by preventing the allergen from reacting with mast cells in the lining of the nose, so preventing the release of histamine and other chemical mediators.

To be effective, anti-allergic drugs should be taken regularly and before an attack occurs. Patients who suffer from hay fever and are allergic to grass pollen should start treatment in early May, before the pollen count becomes high. Those who are allergic to tree pollen should start treatment in February.

Sodium cromoglycate in the form of Rynacrom is particularly useful in the treatment of hay fever. This can be taken in the form of drops, aerosol spray or powder for the nose.

Sodium cromoglycate in the form of Opticrom is very effective in the prevention of allergic conjunctivitis. Antihistamine drugs should not be used in the eyes, as these themselves can give rise to the development of allergy. Steroid eye-drops can lead to glaucoma and damage to the cornea if used to treat conjunctivitis for a prolonged period. Soft contact lenses should not be used while undergoing treatment with Opticrom. A preservative, benzalkonium chloride, used in Opticrom may react adversely with the contact lenses.

The effects of both Rynacrom and Opticrom are short-lived and therefore the dose has to be repeated three to six times a day.

Sodium cromoglycate is useful for mild and moderate hay fever and has no major side effects. It is extremely safe, which makes it particularly useful for children.

Steroids

Steroids, or more correctly corticosteroids, are strong anti-inflammatory drugs that are used to treat many diseases. Many steroids are effective against allergic conditions. Unfortunately, use of steroids in high doses over a long period often gives rise to side effects.

Steroids are used in hay fever when treatment with antihistamine and other drugs has proved not to be effective. They reduce the production of mucus and the swelling of the nasal lining. They are best used to prevent attacks, and it may take some time for the full effect to build up. As in the use of anti-allergic drugs, it is best to start treatment in early May for those allergic to grass pollen and in February for those allergic to tree pollen.

The recent development of steroids that can be used in low doses as nasal sprays and are active only on the lining of the nose and then broken down in the body means that these can be used in the treatment of hay fever with none of the usual associated side effects.

Steroids can be given in the form of a nasal spray or as drops. Both are equally effective, but the latter are preferable when the nasal passages are completely blocked, as they are more likely to penetrate to the affected area. Sprays can be used later, once the swelling has reduced. Care should be taken to administer drops correctly so that they reach the nasal lining and stay in contact there for a few minutes rather than just running down the back of the throat.

Persistent and severe symptoms may require a short course of systemic steroids, such as prednisolone, which is taken in the form of tablets. Steroids in this form have more side effects than those delivered as an aerosol or spray, which rarely enter the bloodstream. Although doctors reluctantly advise steroids in tablet form to treat hay fever, the side effects can be minimised if they are taken for just a week or two at a time. Steroids are very effective in treating hay fever so may be justified in severe cases if used occasionally and sparingly. In some cases, a short course of steroids may be effective in opening up nasal passages so that nasal sprays or drops can be used.

Desensitisation (hyposensitisation; allergen immunotherapy)

This process involves giving injections of a purified allergen extract of progressively increasing concentrations to the allergy sufferer. In some way that is not entirely understood, a person's immune system then becomes *desensitised* to this particular allergen. Reduced levels of antibody and histamine release have been observed in people who have been desensitised. It is also possible that lymphocyte responsiveness to the antigen may be reduced.

Desensitisation, if successful, can offer a cure for allergy rather than just relief of symptoms. However, there are a number of drawbacks to this approach. First, the correct allergen must be identified. This can be difficult, especially where a person is sensitive to a number of different allergens. A mixture of several allergens does not work very well in desensitisation. Secondly, desensitisation seems to work for some people but not for others, and it is impossible to predict in whom it is likely to be successful. Thirdly, some individuals have developed severe reactions to the injected allergen, and in a few cases anaphylactic shock has occurred, resulting in the death of the patient.

Because of the unpredictable outcome of desensitisation and a number of deaths associated with this treatment, it is rarely used as a treatment for allergies.

Perennial rhinitis

In contrast to hay fever, symptoms of perennial rhinitis can occur in varying severity throughout the year. In this form of allergic rhinitis the house dust mite is the principal cause, although mould spores, feathers and animal dander (skin dust) of many species are further causes.

The symptoms are the same as those of hay fever, i.e. a runny nose, watery eyes and sneezing. Other symptoms not involving the nose, such as conjunctivitis, are uncommon. The prolonged nature of this form of rhinitis may lead to several complications:

The sense of smell relies on nerve endings in the nose. When the lining is swollen and the nose is blocked, the sense of smell can be severely reduced. A loss of the sense of smell is a common feature of perennial rhinitis.

Another common complication is the growth of polyps in the nasal passages. These are thickenings of the lining, which grow out into the nasal airways and can block them. Loss of the sense of smell is common among people with polyps, and persistent infection and sinus problems are provoked by them. Polyps can be removed surgically, and often this has to be repeated.

Sinuses are air-filled cavities that are linked to the nose by narrow passages. These can easily get blocked if the nasal lining swells up or if polyps develop. This means that the watery secretions that the sinuses naturally release cannot drain away properly. They may then become infected, produce thick yellow secretions and cause headache, fever and face pain.

Treatment

Treatment for perennial rhinitis is similar to that for hay fever. The first step to take is avoidance of the allergen wherever possible. In cases where house dust is known as, or suspected of being, the prime cause of the condition, steps should be taken to reduce the population of mites and reduce exposure to dust. Details of the sorts of measures to be taken can be found later in this chapter in the section on asthma. Similar measures can be taken to avoid other potential allergens.

Medication, including the use of a combination of antihistamines, decongestants and, in some cases, steroids, may be advised. (*See* treatment section for seasonal rhinitis).

Asthma

Asthma is probably the most common and potentially

serious disorder in which allergy plays an important role. It is the major allergic disease of childhood and is responsible for more absence from school than any other chronic disease. However, the majority of people who suffer from asthma find they have quite mild symptoms, which can be controlled with appropriate medication.

In 1997, the National Asthma Campaign estimated that in the United Kindom about 1 in 25 adults aged 16 and over currently had asthma and 1 in 7 children also suffers from the condition.

Fifty per cent of asthmatics experience their first symptoms before they are five. Asthma is twice as common in boys in this age group as in girls, and they also tend to have more serious symptoms. By the teenage years, new cases of asthma are just as common in girls as in boys, and this pattern continues into adulthood. By the age of 20, the number of new cases has dropped to about half of that occurring in children under five. This decline continues to about age 35, and then the number of new cases begins slowly to increase with age, asthma being then equally common in both sexes.

Asthma can range from being a comparatively mild condition to a very serious illness that can lead to death. In the United Kingdom, 1621 people died from asthma in 1995, 44 fewer than in the previous year. The numbers of people with asthma has been increasing rapidly over the last 20 years. This increase may be partly bercause of better diagnosis but a proportion is also certainly the result of a real increase in the number of people suffering from the condition.

Three times as many children reported an asthma attack in 1992 compared with in 1982. The number of adults consulting their doctor about asthma trebled between 1971 and 1991.

Asthma occurs in almost every country in the world, but the number of people with the condition varies a great deal from country to country. Generally, asthma is more common in the developed world than in the third world, suggesting the importance of some environmental factors. Genetic factors also play an important part in the its development, and it is known to run in families. On the island of Tristan da Cunha in the South Atlantic, over a third of the population suffer from asthma. Because of the isolated geographical position of the island, there has been much inbreeding in the island population, and the majority of the population are descended from the original 15 settlers on the island. Three of these ancestors had asthma. Scientists studying this unique population have recently discovered two faulty genes that make people susceptible to asthma. It is hoped that this discovery will eventually help to identify people at risk. In other ethnic groups, such as the American Indians and the Inuit, asthma is extremely rare.

Asthma can be divided into two main categories:

- *Extrinsic* or *atopic asthma*: this is asthma caused by allergies and is the type that affects most children and

50 per cent of adults. Extrinsic asthma tends to run in families, and it is often associated with other allergic conditions such as eczema and hay fever. Allergy skin tests are usually positive, and the allergen responsible is often easy to identify as symptoms such as wheezing and breathlessness begin shortly after exposure. This form of asthma responds well to treatment.

- *Intrinsic asthma*: this is asthma that is the result of other causes, such as infection, and it is more likely to affect adults. Typically it develops later in life. There is no relation between attacks and exposure to possible allergens, and skin tests prove negative. Attacks are often triggered by colds and chest infections, and treatment is usually less effective.

There is a third category of asthma that is induced by sensitivity to drugs, notably aspirin. Patients with nasal polyps are particularly susceptible.

What is asthma?

Asthma is the sudden and widespread narrowing of the airways (the bronchi) that carry air into the lungs (*see* figure 3.1). When this narrowing occurs, the victim finds it difficult to draw air into the lungs and breathe it out again. All human life needs oxygen to carry out the vital process of respiration, which takes place in the body cells. The bronchi are the branching system of airways that allow the transfer of oxygen from the air we

Figure 3.1: The respiratory system

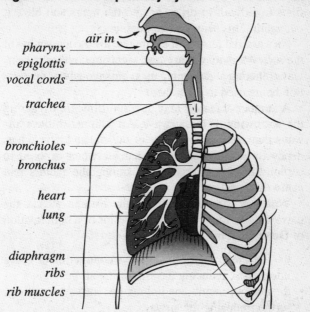

air in

pharynx
epiglottis
vocal cords

trachea

bronchioles
bronchus

heart
lung

diaphragm
ribs
rib muscles

breathe, via the air sacs (alveoli) at their ends, to the bloodstream. The blood then carries the oxygen to where it is needed in the body tissues. The waste product of respiration, carbon dioxide, is carried from the body cells by the bloodstream to the alveoli and from there it is breathed out again via the bronchi.

Normally the bronchi are wide open, and this exchange of gases takes place unnoticed. During an asthmatic attack, the airways are narrowed and the victim finds it difficult to draw air into the lungs and blow it out again. This causes breathlessness.

An essential feature of asthma is that the narrowing of the airways is temporary and reversible, either the airways relaxing and opening up spontaneously or medication being used to relax them.

A number of factors may be responsible for triggering the narrowing of the airways. All asthmatics have airways that are *hyper-reactive* or *twitchy* and have a tendency to go into spasm and narrow when exposed to certain stimuli. Allergens are among the factors that cause this reaction.

Whatever stimulus initiates the asthma attack, the narrowing of the airways is the result of a combination of factors that include:

- the muscle lining of the airways contracting or going into spasm, reducing the size of the air passage.
- the mucous membrane lining t he airway swelling, further reducing the airway.
- an increased mucous secretion from the lining, which cannot be cleared by coughing. This can block the airway completely in some cases.

Recent research has shown that asthma is more than a process that narrows the airways. The persistent inflammation of the linings of the passages is also an important factor. Inflammation leads to a widening and increased leakiness of the blood vessels, causing local

Figure 3.2: Sequence of events in airways in asthma attack

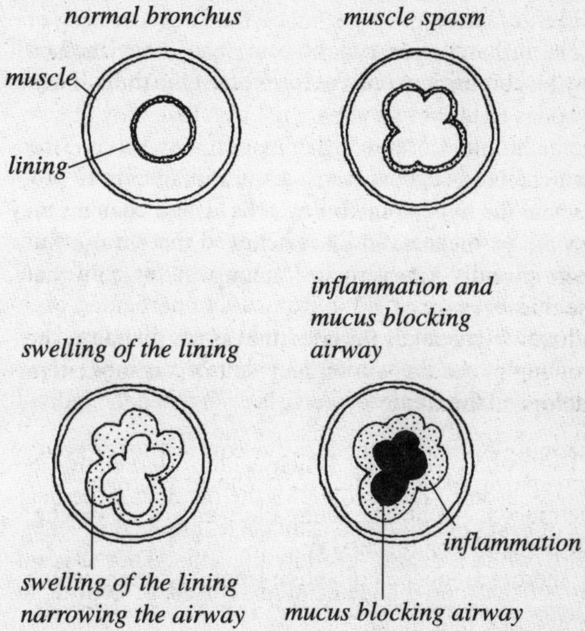

normal bronchus

muscle

lining

muscle spasm

swelling of the lining

inflammation and mucus blocking airway

swelling of the lining narrowing the airway

mucus blocking airway

inflammation

swelling and outpouring of cells of the immune system. This inflammation adds to the narrowing of the air tubes. Inflammation is found to be present in even the mildest of cases.

The inflammation may be acute and short-lived or it may be chronic and present for most of the time. If acute episodes of inflammation are not checked, they may become chronic. Chronic inflammation may lead to structural changes, such as scarring and loss of normal properties of the muscle and lining cells. These changes may become permanent, and it is believed that once asthma becomes fully established, it may last for a lifetime. This has been observed in exposure to particular, occupational allergens. If the condition is not diagnosed early enough, then the worker may develop asthma permanently, and the condition persists even when the individual is removed from workplace exposure.

The same process by which acute inflammation becomes chronic may account for the fact that three-quarters of cases of childhood asthma clear up in the teenage years, while a quarter become life-long. Thus it is important that correct medication is used to control inflammation in asthma.

The allergic reaction is mediated by the mast cells (described in Chapter 1) and is typical of a **Type I** reaction. When an individual is first exposed to a particular allergen, the immune system produces IgE antibody in response. This attaches itself to the mast cells gathered around the lungs and airways. On the next exposure to the same allergen, the antibody combines with the allergen and together they break down the mast cell, releasing a variety of chemicals that cause the allergic reaction. Eosinophils, a type of white blood cell, infiltrate the walls of the airways.

It is characteristic of an asthma attack that breathing out is more difficult than breathing in, so air gets trapped in the lungs. The lungs become over-inflated with air and there is a build-up of carbon dioxide in the lungs and a desire for fresh air.

Symptoms of asthma

The symptoms of asthma can vary greatly in frequency and degree. Some asthmatics are virtually symptom-free with an occasional episode that is mild and brief; others have coughing and wheezing much of the time, with occasional more serious attacks. An attack may come on suddenly within a few minutes or it may build up gradually over days or weeks.

The main symptom of asthma is *shortness of breath*. This can be mild or very severe, and the degree of the breathlessness may also vary according to whether the individual leads a sedentary life or a more active one. In the former case, the shortness of breath may be hardly noticed unless the attack is severe. Others, with more active lives, such as sportsmen and women, may notice any small decrease in their ability to breathe.

Many people first notice their asthma while they are

taking some form of exercise. For children this breathlessness can be particularly disruptive if it prevents par-
ticipation in games at school. Effective medication
means, however, that nowadays asthmatics can participate in sport to the highest levels.

A feeling of *tightness* or *discomfort in the chest* is one
of the first symptoms experienced in an asthmatic attack, and some sufferers may also feel chest pain. There
is difficulty in inhaling deeply because of the lungs being over-inflated and the patient being unable to breathe
out effectively.

Wheezing also accompanies breathlessness and is
caused by vibrations in the narrowed bronchi when air
is forced through them. Wheezing can occur with a
number of other conditions, particularly chest infections, so it does not necessarily confirm that a person is
suffering from asthma.

In very severe asthma attacks, wheezing is usually
present initially but then may disappear altogether. This
can mistakenly be interpreted as the attack easing off.
However, it very often indicates the opposite – that is, a
worsening of the condition as the airways become more
severely blocked and there is a reduction in air flow. At
this stage, the attack is very serious and help must be
given if complete respiratory failure is to be avoided.

In most asthma sufferers, a wheeze disappears completely between attacks but for some a slight one remains permanently.

Cough is a major symptom and is usually worse at

night or in the early morning. Coughing and breathlessness often cause disturbed nights for asthmatics and their families. Why these symptoms get worse at night is not fully understood. It is believed to be because of the natural narrowing of the airways that occurs in everyone. This is not a problem for most people, but in asthmatics, whose airways are already partially constricted, it puts additional strain on their breathing.

For some asthmatics, a dry cough and some wheezing are their only symptoms. The cough is usually dry initially, but as an attack progresses, sputum may be produced, particularly in adults. The sputum is usually colourless unless there is a chest infection present. If this is the case, the cough can be treated with antibiotics, but medication has no effect on a cough associated with asthma. Sometimes the sputum is yellow in colour, but this is not the result of an infection. In this case, the colour is caused by cells of the immune system – eosinophils – which are present in large numbers in allergic reactions.

In more severe episodes of asthma, exhaustion and distress often occur as a result of the effort needed just to breathe. Only a few words can be spoken without a patient gasping for breath. During such an attack, patients will sit with a characteristic upright position or they may lean forward in an effort to help their breathing. They are unlikely to lie down, as this appears to make breathing more difficult. The skin often takes on a blue appearance because of the lack of oxygen in the blood. Shallow, ineffective breathing may follow, and in the most severe cases confusion and lethargy may indicate progressive respiratory failure.

Diagnosis of asthma

Asthma is considered as a possible diagnosis in anyone who wheezes, particularly when episodes start in childhood or early adulthood and are interspersed with periods of complete absence of symptoms. A family history of asthma or allergy is also an important indicator of asthma. Diagnosis of asthma is more difficult when the symptoms first present themselves in adulthood and the symptoms may not be typical, e.g. a cough without wheeze. A number of other disorders may produce wheeze, so it is essential to confirm the diagnosis of asthma with a range of tests to examine lung function and the reversibility of the changes to airways.

A number of devices can be used to measure lung function. The *peak flow meter* measures the speed at which air can be blown out of the lungs. If the airways are restricted, the speed at which air can be blown out is much reduced. If air is blown out as hard as possible, top speed is reached at the beginning . This is called the *peak expiratory flow rate* (PEFR) and is the number of litres of air that would be blown out if the speed could be maintained for a minute. Normal readings range from 350 to 600 litres per minute. During a bad asthma attack, readings can fall as low as 100 litres per minute.

The normal rate will depend on age, sex, height and life-style, and so, for instance, an athlete's peak flow reading would be much higher than that of a similar person who leads a more sedentary lifestyle.

Expiratory flow, other than the peak expiratory flow, can be measured and may be more sensitive to respiratory flow in the more peripheral airways.

Respiratory flow readings in asthmatics vary considerably throughout the day, in contrast to those of normal people in which there is little variation. Among asthmatics, respiratory flow rates are lowest in the late evening and early morning. To confirm a diagnosis of asthma, respiratory flow readings should be taken three times a day for at least a week to demonstrate this variability. The fluctuation in the narrowing of airways is typical of asthma and does not occur in bronchitis. Ideally the readings should be taken in the morning, early afternoon and at night before going to bed. Peak flow readings also give some idea of the severity of asthma and can be used to monitor the effectiveness of medication.

Another device, the *spirometer*, measures vital capacity, i.e. the volume of air that can be expelled from the lungs after a deep breath. The length of time taken to expel the breath is also measured. If lung function is normal, 70 per cent of the vital capacity will be blown out in one second, whereas an asthmatic will expel only 50 per cent, or even as little as 20 per cent, of vital capacity in the same period.

Chest X-rays are useful in the diagnosis of asthma. In

severe cases, X-rays show minor enlargement of the lungs as a result of the decreased ability to expel air from the lungs.

Skin tests are used widely in diagnosing allergic conditions (*see* Chapter 10). Extracts of common allergens are introduced to the skin, using a sterile needle or lance, in order to detect allergic reactions to them.

Levels of IgE antibodies can also be measured. This test alone is not definitive in confirming a diagnosis of asthma as people who are susceptible to a variety of allergens usually have high levels of IgE antibody. However, a positive skin test together with other evidence may confirm the diagnosis.

Bronchial challenge is a procedure that exposes a patient to a potential allergen and then monitors the consequences. The allergic response may be delayed, and so observation continues for at least 48 hours for possible reactions to the allergen. Although this technique is not used widely as a diagnostic tool, it is increasingly used as a measure of the response to drugs and for long-term follow-up. Care has to be taken when using this type of test as it can lead to severe asthmatic attacks. Tests should always be carried out by qualified people with appropriate medical help at hand if needed.

Causes of asthma

As mentioned earlier, there are two main types of asthma, extrinsic and intrinsic. Extrinsic asthma is provoked by allergens and usually develops in childhood, runs in families and is often associated with hay fever and eczema. Intrinsic asthma has little to do with allergy and is the type of asthma that develops in adults. Only 10 per cent of children suffer this type of asthma. This book is primarily concerned with the type of asthma caused by allergies.

Asthma is a condition that has lots of different causes, and each person's asthma will be the result of a combination of both hereditary and environmental factors. Asthma is a condition that runs in families, and some people inherit a genetic predisposition. As mentioned earlier, the gene that causes a person to inherit the tendency has recently been identified. Along with the genetic predisposition, a number of environmental factors are required to ensure that the condition develops. The precise environmental factors are difficult to determine with certainty, but the following factors are known to be significant:

- being brought up in a household where pets are present.
- developing a respiratory infection early on in life.
- being born at the time of year when there are high pollen counts.
- being fed with cow's milk and eggs early on in life.

In addition, certain other factors, known as *adjuvant factors*, increase the chances of getting asthma. These include chemical air pollution and cigarette smoke.

Since there is a range of factors involved, it is difficult to predict exactly which family members will develop the condition.

The development of asthma may be the result of one primary cause, for example an allergy to a pet, but subsequent attacks may be triggered by many different factors, such as exercise, a change in climatic conditions or emotional stress. These factors themselves do not cause an individual to become asthmatic but can provoke an attack once the person has become sensitised.

Essentially, all asthmatics have airways that are hyper-responsive and react to a variety of stimuli that do not have any effect on normal people.

Allergens

Many allergens responsible for causing hay fever also cause asthma, including house dust mites and pollen. The commonest cause of allergic asthma is the house dust mite (*Dermatophagoides pteronyssimus*) or, more precisely, its droppings. The house dust mite lives on moulds and the dead skin cells shed by human bodies. It is found in great concentrations in and around beds, and it is estimated that a bed has around 10,000 mites. Mites are also widely distributed in living areas and thrive in the warm, humid conditions commonly found in British homes.

The house dust mite, although very small, is too big to be inhaled into the nose and lungs. Even the mites' droppings, on which attention is now focused in an attempt to identify precisely the allergen responsible, are too big to be inhaled deep into the lungs. It now seems likely that a substance carried in fragments of the droppings is the allergen that causes asthma.

Many domestic pets, such as dogs, cats, birds, mice, gerbils and hamsters, can cause asthma. Cats are the most likely pet to produce a typical allergic reaction when their dander (tiny particles of skin) is inhaled. Direct contact with the pet may not be necessary as the dander remains in a room long after a pet has been removed and even after the room has been thoroughly cleaned. Cat and dog hair is less likely to be the allergen although dander attached to the hair may provoke an asthmatic reaction.

Pollen
As in hay fever, pollen is recognised as an important cause of asthma. If asthma attacks are seasonal, it is likely that the allergen is a pollen and the exact type may be able to be identified. (*See* Hay Fever).

Moulds and fungi
These are less well-known causes of asthma. They can often cause symptoms when there is no pollen about. Some of these moulds and fungi occur on vegetables and cereal crops.

Occupational allergens
In work environments there are numerous allergenic materials that can cause a range of allergic conditions,

mainly asthma and skin allergies. Asthma can be caused by the inhalation of irritant or allergenic particles or gases from a range of industrial processes, and workers may be exposed to far higher concentrations of these than the general population. Examples of the most common industrial asthma-provoking substances include: various grains, platinum salts, isocyanates, colophony resins in solder, penicillium spores from mouldy cheese, tea powder, green coffee beans, tobacco powder, dyes, various chemicals used in hairdressing, various wood dusts and sawdusts, natural gums, biological enzymes, drugs (especially antibiotics), various paints and solvents, and chromium, nickel and cobalt salts. Over 200 substances have been identified as allergic sensitisers causing occupational asthma. More details on occupational asthma can be found later in the chapter.

Triggers

In addition to the allergens that cause asthma, there are also a number of factors or triggers that can set off or provoke an attack, although in themselves these triggers do not cause a person to become asthmatic. Individuals are sensitive to different triggers. The most common ones are:

- *Exercise*: coughing and wheezing are often brought on by exercise, especially prolonged activity such as jogging. Breathing cold, dry air is also a particularly potent trigger. In both cases, the wheezing results from the cooling and drying of the airways.

- *Infections*: such as the common cold. Asthma often gets worse during a cold, particularly in children, and can persist for several weeks after the infection has disappeared.
- *Emotion*: stress, anxiety, laughing, crying and getting excited can all bring on an attack, particularly in young children.
- *Air temperature and weather conditions*: changes in temperature, particularly going from warm to cold air, can provoke an attack. For others, hot, humid air acts as a trigger.
- *Air pollutants*: pollutants such as car exhaust fumes, cigarette smoke, strong perfumes and aerosols can all be important triggers. Ozone resulting from the action of sunlight on exhaust fumes, together with industrial pollutants such as sulphur dioxide, can all cause serious problems for asthmatics.
- *Drugs*: certain drugs, particularly aspirin, anti-inflammatory painkillers and beta-blockers used for the treatment of high blood pressure, can all provoke attacks in some asthmatics. There are many equally effective alternatives to these drugs which can be used.

Treatment

Asthma can be completely avoided if it is diagnosed accurately, if the correct medication is prescribed and if this is taken regularly. Nowadays, medication is available that can be used to suppress the disease process completely rather than just treat symptoms as they arise. This approach to the treatment of asthma enables the majority of sufferers to lead a full and active life, taking part in all sports and reducing to a minimum the time taken off work or school. Additional medication may be taken if the preventative treatment is not sufficient.

As in all allergic conditions, the first method of treatment should be to avoid the allergen and trigger factors that provoke an attack. Of course, this may not be possible if the allergen has not been identified and, even if it has, it may not be possible to avoid it altogether.

If house dust mites are the cause of asthma, the following measures can be taken to reduce exposure:

- bedding made from artificial materials should be used as these are less attractive to house mites. Duvets and pillows made from feathers and down should be avoided.
- bedding should be cleaned weekly and aired out of doors in sunshine whenever possible.
- curtains, upholstery, mattresses, floors and floor coverings should be vacuumed daily.
- curtains should be washed frequently – every six weeks is recommended.
- a damp duster should be used daily to remove household dust.
- floor boards or linoleum, rather than deep pile carpets, harbour fewer mites.

These measures help to reduce the mite population but will not eradicate them completely.

If a pet is the source of the allergy, consideration should be given to getting rid of it or changing it for another animal that may not have the same effect. Preferably pets should be kept outdoors and certainly never allowed to frequent bedrooms.

During the pollen season, windows and doors should be kept shut, especially on windy, sunny days, to reduce levels within the house. If mould spores are the source of the allergen, steps can be taken to try to eliminate damp from the house. For example, extractor fans in the kitchen and bathroom can reduce condensation.

Factors that are known to trigger asthma attacks should also be avoided. No one should be allowed to smoke in the home, and smoky and polluted environments should be avoided. Asthmatics should stay at home during very severe weather if breathing cold air is likely to bring on an attack. Other triggers, such as emotional upset and infection, may be more difficult to avoid. Although efforts should be made to avoid the factors that trigger an asthma attack, this should not prevent an individual leading a full life. Medication is available that can help in preventing or dealing with the symptoms once they arise.

Medication

As yet there is no cure for asthma, and the use of drugs and medicines are the mainstay of treatment. These work by suppressing or damping down the effects of asthma and have to be taken continuously to be effective.

The primary aim of treatment is to gain complete control of the symptoms by having the bronchi wide open at all times. This means preventing as far as possible acute attacks of asthma as well as the chronic symptoms of wheeze and breathlessness. Most of the medicines currently available can be divided into two groups. The first group works by relieving the muscle spasm so that the bronchi open up. These are taken during an attack to relieve symptoms and are usually effective within 15 minutes. They have no long-term effect on asthma.

The second group of medications works by reducing the inflammation in the airways and so preventing an attack building up. To be effective these need to be taken regularly, even when there are no symptoms. They do not work immediately, but over a period of time they reduce inflammation and stabilise the asthma. They are not effective in attacks.

The medicines in the first group are called *bronchodilators* because they open up the bronchi. They can be divided into three groups:

- *Beta$_2$ stimulants* act by relaxing the smooth muscle of the bronchi. The most commonly prescribed drugs in this group are salbutamol (Ventolin, Aerolin), terbutaline (Bricanyl) and fenoterol (Berotec). They are usually administered as aerosols and are particularly useful in preventing asthma induced by exercise and are often taken before prolonged, strenuous activity. There are two possible side effects – a fine trembling, most noticeable in the hands, and increase in the heart rate when large doses are taken. This does not damage the heart but it may feel uncomfortable.

- *Anticholinergics* tend to be used more in the treatment of chronic bronchitis but have some value in asthma, especially in children under one year old. The commonly prescribed drugs in this group include: oxitropium (Oxivent) and ipratropium (Atrovent). Possible side effects include a dry mouth and blurred vision, and occasionally some patients find difficulty in passing urine and suffer from constipation.

- *Theophylline type* medication can be useful in the management of acute episodes of asthma when used together with the Beta$_2$ group drugs. They are also very useful in the management of nocturnal or night-time asthma.

The second group of preventative drugs includes:

- *Sodium cromoglycate* (*Intal*), which is considered the safest of all drugs to treat asthma and has been available for about 30 years, producing no serious side effects. Sodium cromoglycate appears to act by preventing the release of chemicals from mast cells and reducing hyperactivity in the airways.

   It can be taken as an aerosol and is most useful for preventing mild allergic asthma, particularly in children. It also prevents asthma provoked by exercise. Not everyone responds to it. A few people experience a cough when using it, and children sometimes get a sore, dry throat.

- *Steroids* – when regular use of sodium cromoglycate is not sufficient to control asthma attacks then use of corticosteroids may be considered. These are powerful anti-inflammatory drugs and, when taken in aerosol form, are a safe and effective way of controlling asthma attacks. When used regularly they can reduce spasm and inflammation of the bronchi. Their maximum effect builds up over a period of several weeks. They are not effective once an attack is under way.

  When taken in low doses in the form of an aerosol, very little of the steroid reaches the bloodstream, and there are few side effects. The most commonly prescribed aerosol steroids are beclomethasone (Aerobec, Becotide) or budesonide (Pulmicort). A low dose is regarded as up to 400 micrograms a day. The only side effects of these steroids taken in low doses are hoarseness and oral thrush (a fungal infection that may show up as a red rash with white spots in the mouth and at the back of the throat). Both these side effects can be overcome by a more effective delivery of the drug using a spacer device (*see* next section). At higher doses, inhaled steroids may cause children's growth to slow down temporarily. In adults there may be a risk of thinning of the bones (osteoporosis).

Treatment with steroids in tablet form is used only when all other treatments have failed. They are nearly always very effective against severe asthma and are now usually used in short, sharp bursts for severe, sudden attacks that do not respond to inhaler aerosols. Short courses of steroid tablets, such as prednisolone, taken for two weeks or less, three or four times a year, are not thought to cause significant side effects.

A small number of people have severe asthma that does not respond to any other treatment, and they have to take steroids on a long-term basis. The risks of possible side effects are higher in this group. Possible side effects include high blood pressure, diabetes, indigestion, weight gain, muscle weakness and weakening of the bones (osteoporosis). Steroids must not be stopped suddenly, as long-term use of steroids prevents the adrenal gland making the normal amounts of cortisol – a steroid hormone.

Although the side effects of treatment can be serious, they have to be weighed up against the consequences of severe asthma attacks, which can be, at best, very debilitating and disruptive and, at worst, fatal.

Devices used to take asthma medications

A number of devices have been developed to enable drugs used in the treatment of asthma to be delivered directly to the lungs. Inhalation of drugs in an aerosol or powder form is a more effective way of taking medication than tablets. The drug is able to reach the lungs directly. Smaller doses can be taken and therefore possible side effects are reduced.

Medication in the form of syrup is often given to infants who are unable to use inhalers. Tablets may be preferred by some asthmatics, particularly if they have trouble with asthma at night. Slow-release tablets of bronchodilators such as Ventolin and Bricayle can be taken at night to prevent attacks in the early morning.

At least a dozen different inhalers are now available. Some suit some people more than others. Most have been developed by drug companies for their own products, and so not all the devices are available for all medications.

Metered dose inhalers are the most common form of inhalers, and most asthma medications are available in this form. Basically this device consists of a pressurised canister that releases a cloud of the drug when pressed. Correct technique in using this inhaler is essential. The patient breathes out and the aerosol must be released just as a breath is being taken in so that the maximum amount of aerosol reaches the lungs. Good coordination is needed to use it properly, so it may not be suitable for all asthmatics, for example, young children and those with arthritic hands.

The *Volumatic* is a device that fits on to a metered dose inhaler. With this attached, there is no need to coordinate the firing of the inhaler so more of the drug is delivered to the lungs rather than the mouth. The disadvantage of the volumatic is its size, which makes it less convenient to carry around.

The *autoinhaler* is a breath-actuated metered dose inhaler. It is easy to use as it releases the drug automatically on the intake of breath. Coordination is less important as the medication is always released at the right time.

The *Diskhaler* delivers the drug in a powder form rather than in an aerosol form. Some people find the taste of the powder form preferable. It is also breath-actuated and therefore easy to use. It is also possible to monitor exactly how many doses have been used, which is not possible with many of the other devices.

The *Turbohaler* is another breath-actuated dry powder device. It is very easy to use, and its small size makes it convenient to carry around. The amount of powder in each dose is small, and so it is less likely to cause coughing than devices such as the *Diskhaler.* The number of doses taken cannot be monitored, but an indicator shows when the device is almost empty.

Nebulisers are machines that turn a liquid medication into a fine mist that can be inhaled in much higher doses than can be obtained through any of the devices mentioned above. They are used to treat patients with very severe asthma. Nebulisers are found in hospitals and some GP practices, and patients with prolonged severe asthma may keep a machine at home. Care must be taken when using these machines.

Nebulisers are also sometimes employed to treat

young children as they require little cooperation to be used effectively.

Occupational asthma

Exposure to allergic sensitisers in the workplace is very common, and occupational asthma accounts for 2 per cent of all adult asthma. Over 1000 new cases occur every year.

There are well over 200 substances used in industrial processes that are recognised as causes of industrial asthma. The most common groups of industrial allergens and the processes in which they are used are listed below:

- isocyanates – used for making plastic foam, synthetic inks, paints, adhesives and electronic component insulation
- platinum salts – used in platinum refining and found in laboratories
- acid anhydride and amine hardening agents – used for making adhesives, plastics, moulding resins and surface coatings
- soldering flux fumes from resin – used in the electronics industry
- enzymes in biological washing powders, baking, brewing – used in the food, fish and leather industries
- grain, meal or flour dust (barley, oats, rye, wheat or maize) found on farms (including contaminants of

flour such as weevils) – used in the baking and milling industries

• drugs, especially antibiotics, cimetidine and piperazine

Some of these substances are more liable to bring on asthma than others. Bakers' flour has been known to cause asthma since ancient times and is a potent allergen. It is not only the flour that can cause the allergic reaction but contaminants within it, including mites, fungal spores and finely chopped wheat hairs. About 20 per cent of bakers exposed to wheat flour develop asthma.

Up to 50 per cent of workers exposed to platinum salts develop asthma, and there are strict regulations governing the working conditions of those who may be exposed to them. Anyone who is found to be sensitive to these salts by skin-prick testing is excluded from employment involving these substances.

Asthma is likely to develop in 50 per cent of workers exposed to protein-splitting enzymes and about 10 per cent of those working with toluene di-isocyanate. Asthma is also common in workers exposed to wood dust, particularly that from Canadian red cedar, South African boxwood, oak and mansonia. Up to 1 in 20 workers exposed to these dusts develops asthma.

Anhydrides are one of the most potent groups of industrial allergens, particularly phthalic acid anhydride and trimellitic anhydride. These are used as hardening agents to set epoxy resins. Once IgE antibody levels to these substances have built up on initial exposure, further encounters with them leads to an allergic response developing within minutes. In addition to asthma, hay fever, muscle pain, high temperatures and anaemia may also develop.

A number of people are exposed to some of these substances in the course of pursuing their hobbies, do-it-yourself and leisure activities. Exposure in these circumstances is not regulated, and people may be at greater risk than if they come into contact with these substances during the course of their work.

Unlike most of the causes and triggers of asthma already discussed, many of the reactions to these allergens are delayed. Patients generally complain of shortness of breath, chest tightness, wheezing and cough, often in association with symptoms such as sneezing and watery eyes. Symptoms may develop during working hours in association with a specified dust or gas, but often they do not arise for several hours after leaving work. This may make the association with a particular substance difficult to determine. The symptoms often disappear at weekends and during holidays. However, in some cases the asthma may become permanent, especially if the link is not made between the condition and exposure to the particular allergen causing it and protective measures are not taken soon enough.

Diagnosis and treatment of occupational asthma are similar to those for other forms of asthma. Employers have a legal duty to protect their employees from hazards in the workplace, including the development of allergies. Risks from occupational asthma can be reduced by, for example, suppressing dust in industries in which allergens have been identified or using effective protective clothing. Elimination of exposure to all allergens may not always be possible. If a person is susceptible, he or she should be removed from exposure altogether.

Allergic pneumonia

Some allergic reactions can affect the tissue of the lung itself rather than the airways. This produces a pneumonia-like illness, called allergic pneumonia in the United States. In the United Kingdom it is known as *allergic alveolitis*, emphasising the involvement of the alveoli. The major symptom, not surprisingly, is breathlessness.

Allergic pneumonia can be caused by an allergic response after inhalation of considerable amounts of a micro-organism or a foreign animal or vegetable protein. Less commonly, simple chemicals may also be responsible for causing the condition.

The best-known of these diseases is 'farmer's lung', which is associated with repeated inhalation of dust from hay containing the micro-organism *Micropolyspora faeni*. This microscopic fungus grows rapidly in damp mouldy hay, and its growth causes the hay to heat up, sometimes to a temperature of 50–60°C. When the hay is moved as feed or bedding for livestock, millions of the spores of the fungus are liberated into the air. The farmer breathes in the spores, and because of their very small size, they are able to reach the distant air sacs (alveoli) at the end of the airways. The spores stick to the walls of the air sacs and produce the allergic reaction. The flu-like symptoms of aching joints, high fever, coughing and breathlessness do not appear for several hours, usually in the evening. By morning all the symptoms have gone, but the process starts again when the farmer returns to the same work. If exposed to these conditions over a prolonged period, permanent damage may result. The farmer suffers from severe shortness of breath and is unable to work. It is a recognised industrial disease. The introduction of modern farming methods, especially the use of storage silos, has led to a reduction in the number of people sufferers.

There are a number of other allergic pneumonias associated with occupations in which workers are exposed to a large number of micro-organisms. Some of these are listed in Table 3.1, with the source of the particles.

A disease with symptoms identical to farmer's lung can arise in individuals who work in buildings in which the environment is controlled by air-conditioners and humidifiers. This condition is referred to as 'humidifier fever', and it can arise in anyone working in a building in which recycled water is used to humidify the air. The tanks that store the water can readily become contaminated with a wide range of microscopic living organisms which have been found to be responsible for causing humidifier fever. The problem can be cured by rais-

Table 3.1: Selected causes of allergic alveolitis (allergic pneumonia)

Disease	Antigen	Source of particle
Farmer's lung	*Micropolyspora faeni* *Thermoactinomyces vulgaris*	Mouldy hay
Pigeon fancier's lung	Serum proteins and droppings	Pigeons
Air-conditioner (or humidifier) lung	*M. faeni, T. vulgaris*	Humidifiers and air conditioners
Cheesewasher's lung	*Penicillium sp.*	Mouldy cheese
Malt worker's lung	*Aspergillus fumigatus* or *A. clavatus*	Mouldy barley, malt
Coffee worker's lung	Coffee bean dust	Coffee beans
Chemical worker's lung	Isocyanates, phthalic anhydride, vinyl chloride	Manufacturing of polyurethane foam, moulding, insulation, meat wrapping

ing the temperature of the water or adding disinfectant. However, the latter course of action may contribute to other symptoms which have been called 'sick building syndrome'.

Pigeon fancier's lung is another allergic pneumonia that can arise in people who keep pigeons. This condition is the result of inhalation of dried bird droppings and the fine powdery 'bloom' that covers the feathers. The main symptoms of this disease, which usually arise several hours after handling the pigeons, are chills, coughing and breathlessness. If the disease is recognised early enough, a complete cure is possible if the hobby is given up. About a quarter of pigeon fanciers show evidence of some sort of allergy to the bird but not all suffer the symptoms of allergic pneumonia.

A similar condition can arise in those who keep budgerigars as pets. This condition, which is very rare, is known as 'budgerigar fancier's lung'. The disease results from the inhalation of dried particles from budgerigar droppings and mainly affects the person responsible who cleans the cages.

Only a small proportion of those exposed to the allergen are likely to develop symptoms, and usually after prolonged exposure to the antigen. Continuous or frequent low-level exposure to the antigen may result in permanent damage to the lung tissue.

Individuals with a history of previous allergic disease such as hay fever and asthma are no more likely to develop this type of condition than anyone else.

4

Allergies of the Eye and Ear

Allergy and the eye

The eye is a unique organ in the body in that it cannot mount an allergic response. The eye itself has very few blood vessels, and few mast cells are found in the eye. As the eye cannot employ the usual immunological defence mechanisms used by other parts of the body, it has a structure that goes some way towards defending itself from invading organisms. The cornea, the transparent part of the eye in front of the lens, comprises cells that are packed very closely together, preventing particles, including bacteria and allergens, from entering the eye. Another protective mechanism is the production of tears, which, together with blinking, help to keep the eye clean. Tears contain a powerful disinfectant called lysosome and also antibodies, mainly IgA, that react with and neutralise allergens and bacteria.

The conjunctiva is a delicate mucous membrane that covers the white part of the eye and lines the inside of both the upper and lower eyelids. This membrane is well served with blood capillaries and is very sensitive to a range of allergens. There are numerous mast cells in the conjunctiva, and it can readily become inflamed. When this happens, the blood supply to the conjunctiva increases and the eye looks red. Tears are secreted in an attempt to wash away the offending substance, causing the eyes to run. Particles that accumulate in the inner corner of the eye cause irritation and are removed by rubbing the eyes. Despite the various mechanisms designed to protect the eye from offending particles, sometimes allergens from the atmosphere enter the eye and elicit an allergic response. The most common of these reactions is *allergic conjunctivitis* (inflammation of the conjunctiva).

Figure 4.1: The eye

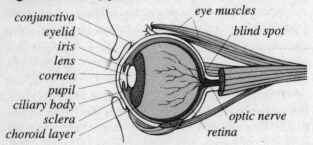

conjunctiva
eyelid
iris
lens
cornea
pupil
ciliary body
sclera
choroid layer

eye muscles
blind spot

optic nerve
retina

Allergic conjunctivitis

This condition commonly arises as part of a larger allergic syndrome, e.g. hay fever, but it can also occur alone through direct contact with airborne substances such as pollen, fungal spores, dusts and animal danders.

Symptoms of this condition include extreme itchiness, particularly of the inner corners of the eye, where the allergen particles have accumulated. The eyes become red and there may be excessive watering. The conjunctiva may swell up, and in severe cases the eye may close altogether. The itchiness of this condition often makes rubbing the eye irresistible. This , however, relieves the condition for only a short time and usually leads to further swelling and redness.

The itchiness associated with this condition indicates that it is caused by an allergic response. In contrast, if the eyes become sore or painful it indicates that infection is more likely to be the cause. The presence on the eyelashes of a thick mucus and crusted material that cause the eyes to stick together on waking confirms that an infection is present.

Allergic conjunctivitis can be caused by the same sort of airborne allergens that cause hay fever, such as grass, tree or flower pollens, dusts and moulds. It can also be caused by sensitivity to cosmetics, proprietary eye preparations, tobacco smoke and chemicals. The condition may also be the result of reactions to food and food additives, such as artificial colourings. Occasionally, allergic conjunctivitis may be the only symptom of food allergy.

The eye is more likely to be involved in hay fever (seasonal rhinitis) than in cases of perennial rhinitis

caused by, for example, allergy to the house dust mite.
Nevertheless, allergic conjunctivitis can occur as a consequence of allergy to pets and may be troublesome in
children.

Vernal conjunctivitis

This is a more serious, although very rare, form of conjunctivitis which involves the undersurface of the eyelids. It is most common in males between the ages of
five and twenty, and boys are three times more likely to
suffer from it than girls. There is evidence that vernal
conjunctivitis is an atopic disorder, that is, it is more
likely to occur in individuals who have an hereditary
tendency to develop allergies. The word 'vernal' comes
from the Latin *vernalis*, which means 'spring', but the
condition can occur throughout the year. However, the
disease often flares up in the spring, causing severe
symptoms. The condition may be short-lived or it can
last for several months.

The main symptoms of vernal conjunctivitis are redness of the eye and severe itching, as in allergic conjunctivitis, but, in addition, there is a thick, heavy discharge and an intolerance of light (photophobia). The
most distinctive feature of the disease is the appearance
of square, hard, wart-like protuberances inside the upper eyelid. These are usually pale pink to greyish in colour and produce a cobblestone effect on the inside of the
eyelid. In the most severe cases the cornea may be in-

volved, causing pain and increased sensitivity to light. These 'warts' can heal, but in prolonged cases there may be some permanent scarring of the cornea. The symptoms usually disappear during the cold months. The condition usually becomes milder over the years and often resolves itself after five to ten years.

Treatment

The allergen, whether it has been identified or is just suspected as causing the condition, should be avoided. Frequent use of a bland eyewash such as a weak saline solution can be used to reduce irritation. Contact lenses should not be worn.

The use of sodium cromoglycate in the form of eye drops (Opticrom) may also be helpful, particularly to prevent development of the symptoms when exposure to the allergen is expected.

Oral antihistamines, i.e. taken by mouth, may also help the condition. Topical antihistamines are also available, but care should be taken if using these as the preparations themselves or, more particularly, the pre-servatives used in them can cause an allergic response. As most people respond equally well or better to oral antihistamines it is probably wiser to stick to those.

In more serious conditions topical steroids may be used as a last resort to counteract itching and intoler-ance of light. These steroids should only be used for the minimum period when the symptoms are active as they may be potentially dangerous. Intraocular pressure, that is, blood pressure within the eye, should be measured regularly during treatment with steroids.

Allergies and the ears

Serous otitis media is a common ear disorder in children and is the inflammation of the middle ear with the formation of fluid. Sometimes this fluid is very thick and sticky and gives rise to a condition known as *glue ear*.

The middle ear is an air-filled cavity between the eardrum and the skull. Its function is to transmit vibrations from the eardrum to the brain. A channel, the Eustachian tube, runs from the back of the nose to the middle ear and keeps the cavity supplied with air. The middle ear is

Figure 4.2: The ear

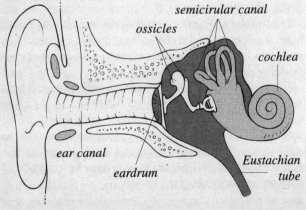

semicirular canal

ossicles

cochlea

ear canal

eardrum

Eustachian tube

normally ventilated three to four times a minute as the Eustachian tube opens during swallowing, chewing or yawning. This equalises the air pressure between the ears and the throat. The Eustachian tube can become blocked in some circumstances. The blockage may be caused by the inflammation of the tissues in the surrounding area, enlargement of the adenoids or benign or malignant growths in or near the tube. In some cases it may be an allergic response that causes the inflammation and the swelling that blocks the tube. The precise steps in the development of this condition are uncertain, but it seems likely that allergy plays a part in at least some cases of serous otitis media. In particular, food allergy is thought to be a contributing factor.

In children the Eustachian tube is very narrow, only about 1 mm wide, and can easily get blocked with the thick glue-like material. Deafness may result as the blocked tube interferes with the transmission of sound waves. Glue ear is the commonest form of deafness in childhood and may cause problems with schooling and/ or delay the development of speech.

Treatment with antihistamines can relieve Eustachian tube obstruction when the cause is allergic. In the other cases, where the cause is bacterial, antibiotics may be useful. In some cases a surgical procedure is needed to unblock the Eustachian tube to allow air into the middle ear. The tonsils and adenoids may also be removed if they are greatly enlarged.

5

Skin Allergies

The skin is the largest organ of the body. It serves several important functions, including protecting the body against infection by bacteria, viruses and parasites, regulating water loss and alerting a person to changes in the external environment, such as fluctuations in temperature. It acts as the body's primary barrier against the outside world, and so it is not surprising that it is subject to a number of allergies.

There is a lot of confusion in the way that different skin conditions are named. The word *dermatitis* simply means 'inflammation of the skin' but is often used as a shorthand term to refer to allergic *contact dermatitis*. This is an allergic condition that results from a reaction to a substance in contact with the skin.

Another form of dermatitis, *atopic dermatitis*, is more commonly known as *eczema*, but sometimes this too is just referred to as dermatitis. Eczema, or atopic dermatitis, often occurs in people who are subject to a number of allergies, that is, they have an inherited predisposition for these conditions. The most usual associated allergies are hay fever and asthma. When both parents have eczema, there is a greater than 50 per cent chance that their children will also develop the condition.

Eczema (atopic dermatitis)

Eczema is a very common skin condition that causes a reddish rash (dark if the skin is brown or black) which can be very itchy and causes flaking of the skin. In severe cases, the skin may also crack and weep.

Eczema is generally considered to be a childhood condition, although older children and adults may also develop it. About three-quarters of affected children show signs of eczema before they are a year old, and the majority of them will grow out of it by the time they reach adulthood.

Eczema can be classified according to the timing of the onset of the disease:

- *Infantile eczema* typically starts between the ages of two and six months and is more common in bottle-fed than breast-fed babies. The rash develops initially on the face and then progresses to the trunk, arms and legs. The rash is red in colour and initially it may be quite mild. Increasing redness is an indication that the condition is getting worse. The baby may rub his or her face in order to relieve the itching. Many of the children who develop eczema at this early stage of life will be clear of the condition within a few years.

- *Childhood eczema* develops in the toddler years, from eighteen months onwards. In this form of eczema, the rash typically settles in the creases inside the arms and at the back of the legs, which are known as the flexor surfaces of the body. The wrists, ankles and fingers are also commonly affected. Small fluid-filled blisters, called 'vesicles', may develop on the skin. These weep and in some cases may bleed if scratched. Crusts may then develop on the skin. Crusting and cracking of the skin are particularly prominent in this age group.

  Eczema can be very distressing in school-age children when fellow pupils make fun of the appearance of the skin. It may also cause problems when it is mistakenly thought to be a contagious condition. This is not the case. Most people who develop eczema as young children will grow out of it by the onset of puberty.

- *Adult eczema.* Eczema is less common in adults. At this stage of onset, eczema typically affects the skin folds, such as the eyelids, the forehead, around the mouth, knees, elbows, wrists and fingers. It also commonly affects the hairline on the scalp. The skin lesions tend to be thick and crusty, with blisters lying under the skin (papules). Eczema may lie dormant for several years and then flare up again, particularly when an individual is under emotional stress. This form of eczema may be very localised, for example on the lips or nipples.

The causes of eczema

The exact cause of eczema remains a mystery. Patients usually have high levels of IgE antibody and elevated concentrations of eosinophils, but it is not clear what their significance is in this disease. One theory suggests that eczema is a result of contact between damaged skin and allergens from the house dust mite or domestic pets. Diet is also believed to be important.

Eczema has a strong relationship with other allergic conditions but the exact connection is unclear. About 50 per cent of children with eczema also have hay fever or asthma. In addition, about 60 per cent of children with asthma also have eczema. It is not uncommon for children who suffer from both conditions to find that when the eczema is particularly severe, they have little trouble with their asthma, and vice versa.

Eczema runs in families and is more common in children of allergic parents.

It is thought that allergy to certain foods could be a major cause of eczema in both children and adults. The most common cause of the condition in babies is cow's milk. Eggs may also be important. Babies who are breast-fed are less likely to develop the condition, and exclusive and prolonged breast-feeding can delay and, in some cases, prevent the disease. This protective effect of human breast milk is thought to be because of the presence of IgA antibody in the milk as well as a factor that accelerates further production of this antibody. Some studies show that babies with eczema have lower levels of IgA than babies who do not. As well as helping prevent the development of eczema in babies, breast-feeding is also thought to provide some protection against other allergies in later life.

Babies who are going to develop the disease do so usually in the first two months of life. If breast-feeding is not possible and the baby is thought to be at risk, then one of the soya-based milk products can be used. If there is a family history of eczema, then it may be wise to avoid cow's milk entirely in the first year. Some babies may be very sensitive to cow's milk and egg protein, and it is possible that the cow's milk and egg protein in the mother's diet is enough to cause eczema in the baby. A mother who is breast-feeding and has even slight allergic tendencies may consider avoiding cow's milk and eggs in her own diet. In some cases a baby may not show sensitivity to cow's milk and eggs while being breast-fed but may go on to develop symptoms when these are introduced into the diet directly. However, the exclusion of cow's milk and egg protein is not the whole story, as even when all these preventive measures are taken some babies still go on to develop eczema.

Some studies have shown that if eggs and cow's milk are totally excluded from the diet, eczema in very young children will improve in the majority of cases, but in others, there will be little or no improvement.

Cow's milk may also be a cause of eczema in older children and adults. It is also likely that a number of other known food allergens such as wheat, eggs, fish, cheese, citrus fruit and nuts may also cause eczema in some people. Eczema may get worse when spicy foods, alcohol and certain food dyes and colourings, such as tartrazine, are eaten.

Factors that exacerbate eczema

Flare-ups of eczema are unpredictable, and it can be very difficult to pinpoint a reason why the condition suddenly gets worse and then, for no apparent reason, improves again. Exposure to many of the factors that cause eczema may be responsible for making eczema worse, but the course and nature of the condition varies and different people are affected by particular triggers. The following are a list of some of the factors that may exacerbate the condition:

- *Chemicals* – the chemicals used in modern washing powders can often cause problems for eczema sufferers. Clothes washed in these can cause flare-ups in the condition. A sudden worsening of the condition can sometimes be traced back to a change of washing powder or alteration in the formulation by the manufacturers. The change to biological washing powders in the 1980s caused a big increase in eczema.

  Similarly, chemical constituents of soaps, shampoos, washing-up liquids and skin creams and lotions may aggravate an existing condition. Excessive use of soap and bathing can cause drying and irritation of the skin.

- *Stress* – although eczema is a stressful condition in itself, stress and anxiety can often make it worse.
- *Clothing* – both wool and nylon are possible irritants and can cause eczema to flare up. Wool, which is rough on the skin, may also contain natural lanolin which can be an irritant. Clothing with stiff, hard or rough edges may aggravate the condition. Loose, cotton clothing is preferable for anyone with eczema.
- *Diet* – as already mentioned, a number of foods are suspected of causing eczema. The same foods are also probably responsible for provoking a flare-up of the condition in susceptible people. A restricted diet often helps improve eczema. Cow's milk, eggs and chicken are the first items to be removed if diet is to be restricted. If such a diet is going to help, improvement shows within six weeks.
- *Season* – sufferers from eczema often find that the condition gets worse in cold weather.
- *Other allergens* – the prime culprit in precipitating eczema is the house dust mite. Precautions should be taken, as described in the chapter on asthma, to reduce the population of house dust mites within the home. Pets can also exacerbate the condition.
- *Infections* – skin infections or coughs and colds may provoke attacks, particularly in children.

Treatment
As in every allergic condition, if the offending allergen is known all contact with it should be avoided. This may

include removing household pets, which often cause eczema in children. Reducing exposure to the house dust mite may also be helpful. Where a food is suspected as the source of the allergen an exclusion diet may be tried. The foods most commonly associated with provoking eczema are dairy products made from cow's milk, eggs, chicken and sometimes wheat. All these products can be excluded from the diet and then reintroduced one at a time. In this way it may be possible to determine which one is responsible for the condition. This food can then be excluded from the diet permanently.

A variety of ointments and creams are available to soothe and relieve the symptoms of eczema. Whether a preparation is applied as a cream or an ointment is largely a matter of personal preference. An ointment tends to be greasier than a cream, and some people find them easier to apply sparingly and accurately. Creams tend to be absorbed more quickly by the skin. Some people prefer to use an emollient as a cream, as it is applied more liberally, along with a steroid in the form of an ointment, which must be targeted more carefully to a specific area. Some newer preparations combine the qualities of creams and ointments in that they are greasier and more water protective than creams but wash off readily.

- *Corticosteroid creams and ointments* – these are the most effective treatments for eczema and can be applied directly to the affected area as a cream or ointment. They should be used sparingly, however, as they have a number of side effects and they are also expensive. Some weaker steroid creams, such as hydrocortisone 1 per cent, are relatively safe and can be bought over the counter without a prescription. These can be used for a short time if the eczema gets particularly bad. If this treatment does not improve the condition, stronger steroid cream can be prescribed by a doctor. This is prescribed in the minimum strength necessary and only for the length of time needed for an improvement.

The side effects of steroid creams when used over a long period or in large amounts on the skin include reddening and thinning, which may be irreversible. Stretch marks may appear, and acne and additional hair growth may also occur. These side effects are particularly marked when creams and ointments are used on the face. Only very mild steroid creams (hydrocortisone 0.5 per cent) should be used to treat facial eczema. In children, the prolonged and widespread use of high potency steroid creams and ointments should be avoided as the use of such drugs can affect the body's own production of steroids. This can lead to a deficiency in hormones and a reduction in growth. This is very rare but great caution should nonetheless be exercised.

New steroid creams have been developed that are less likely to produce such serious side effects as they are not so readily absorbed into the skin as the older type of preparations. Mometasone furoate (brand name Elocon) and fluticasone propionate (brand name Cutivate) are two of the new generation of steroid creams.

- *Emollient creams and ointments* are particularly useful in dry, eczematous conditions. They can be rubbed liberally into the skin on the face and body several times a day. This treatment moisturises and smooths the skin and relieves itching. They can be rubbed into the skin instead of scratching. Emollients are often used intermittently with steroids, as prolonged use of steroids is not advised (*see* above).

- *Aqueous creams and emulsifying ointments* are popular treatments to help relieve symptoms. Some of these contain wool fat and related substances, including lanolin, which can themselves cause allergic reactions. One of the most widely used and safest is called *aqueous cream*, which contains an emulsifying ointment with phenoxyethanol in freshly boiled and cooled purified water. Modern ointments prevent water getting on to the eczematous area. They usually consist of soft paraffin and have a mild anti-inflammatory effect.

- *Bathing* – the skin of most people suffering from eczema is very dry and dry skin tends to be thin and more itchy than normal skin. Scratching such thin skin can cause damage and can make the eczema worse. Taking regular baths can help in relieving the symptoms of eczema in some people as long as the water is not too hot. The use of bath oils can help the skin become less dry and therefore not so itchy. Baths of short duration are advisable, as staying in the bath too long tends to dry out the skin. Soaps and bubble baths should be avoided as these can also cause the skin to dry. The use of emollient creams that soften and moisturise the skin are particularly effective if they are used within minutes of having a bath while the skin is still warm and soft. Soft skin is less prone to damage when scratched.

- *Ultraviolet light* is known to have a beneficial effect on eczema. A holiday in a warm, sunny climate can often help to clear up the condition. A course of treatment called *psoralen plus ultraviolet light A*, or PUVA, can be used to control severe outbreaks of eczema in older people. This treatment consists of taking a plant extract, known as psoralen, by mouth and about two hours later sitting under a source of high intensity ultraviolet light. If this treatment is continued over a long period the side effects are the same as over-exposure to natural sunlight, that is, premature ageing of the skin and possible development of skin cancers. Because of the side effects, it is only recommended as a means of getting the condition under control and not as a long-term treatment. For the same reason it is not used in children or young adults.

- *Antihistamines* – itching can become much worse at night-time, especially while in bed, when the body may become overheated. Antihistamines are often prescribed for children to take at night as a sedative to reduce scratching. Antihistamines without a sedative effect for daytime use may also be prescribed.

* *Short fingernails* – fingernails should be kept short to avoid damage from scratching, which can break the skin and introduce infection.
* *Antibiotics* – normal, healthy skin presents an effective barrier to the bacteria that naturally inhabit the surface of the skin. Damaged and inflamed skin is much more likely to become infected with bacteria, in particular *Staphylococcus*. Antibiotics are prescribed to clear up such infections.

Complications of eczema

A potentially serious complicating infection is that caused by the herpes group of viruses, which are responsible for causing cold sores and chicken pox. Contact with this virus should be avoided wherever possible. If a member of the family has a cold sore, it should be covered to prevent the eczema sufferer from coming in contact with it. This virus can be responsible for a super-imposed rash, resembling the blistering of eczema. In addition, there is a sudden worsening of the condition with increased blistering, and the child may feel unwell and feverish. In rare cases, the virus can reach internal organs. Medical help should be sought immediately and a drug called acyclovir (brand name Zovirax) can be given, which can prevent the viral infection from spreading further.

Contact dermatitis

Contact dermatitis is a skin rash that occurs as result, as
its name suggests, of contact with an external agent. The
rash looks exactly like the rash that occurs with eczema
(allergic dermatitis), but it can occur anywhere on the
body where there has been contact with the offending
material. Not all contact dermatitis is caused by an allergy; many cases result from some chemical irritant.

- *Irritant dermatitis* – irritants may damage normal
  skin or exacerbate an existing dermatitis. With weak
  irritants, e.g. soap, detergents or even water, several
  days' exposure may be necessary to cause recognisa-
  ble clinical changes in the skin. Stronger irritants
  such as acids and alkalis can cause visible changes in
  the skin almost immediately. The mechanisms by
  which these irritants damage the skin is as yet unknown.

  Irritant dermatitis frequently occurs in domestic
  situations, and the hands are often the parts of the
  body that are affected. Frequent use of water, detergents and other cleaning agents causes the skin to lose
  natural oils and moisture, leading to drying and
  cracking. The severity of the condition depends on
  how often the hands are immersed in water. The problem often starts under a ring, where detergent or soap
  can lodge. The condition then typically spreads to affect the thin skin at the side of the fingers, the webs

between them and the back of the hands. In very severe cases the palms may also be affected.

Irritant dermatitis is also common in workplaces where solvents are used to remove grease from metal surfaces. These solvents work equally well at removing natural oils and moisture from the skin.

The problem of irritant dermatitis can often be solved by wearing protective gloves when undertaking such work. However, a number of people have found that they are allergic to protective gloves, particularly those containing latex. In recent years, allergy to latex gloves has become a serious problem in the Health Service where they are used routinely for many procedures. It appears that the starch that is used to line the gloves to make them easier to put on acts as a carrier for latex. In one or two severe cases, anaphylactic reactions have resulted from allergy to protective gloves. Other types of gloves are available that may not cause such problems.

- *Allergic contact dermatitis* this form of contact dermatitis is a delayed hypersensitivity reaction. It is not the same sort of allergic response as that involved in other conditions, such as hay fever, asthma or even eczemas, which are Type I reactions (*see* Chapter 1). That responsible for allergic contact dermatitis is a Type IV reaction and does not involve antibodies. The response occurs when certain materials in contact with the skin react with proteins within the skin to form an allergen. Some people then produce a hypersensitive reaction to this allergen. Atopic individuals are at no greater risk from this form of contact dermatitis than those who do not generally suffer from allergies.

It takes between six and ten days to become sensitised to strong substances such as poison ivy and up to several years of repeated and prolonged exposure for weaker ones. Following sensitisation, re-exposure to the material may bring about itching and dermatitis within four to twelve hours. People often find it difficult to believe that they have become allergic to substances they have used for years.

Diagnosis of contact dermatitis

Diagnosis of contact dermatitis is usually not difficult, especially if the patient is seen shortly after the symptoms have developed. Initially, the rash is usually concentrated in the area where the skin has been in contact with the offending material, for example where a watchstrap or necklace has been worn. In severe cases, the rash may spread to cover many areas of the body. The condition may increase in severity over several days, even though there is no further contact with the substance concerned. If the rash is on the hands, diagnosis may be more difficult as the hands are in contact with a variety of substances throughout the day.

Patch tests can be a reliable method of identifying the contactant as they reproduce the conditions that caused the skin disorder in the first place. For this reason, a patch test should never be undertaken during an acute phase of the disease in case the condition is exacerbated.

Patch testing is usually carried out on intact skin on the back. Small amounts of the suspect substances, dissolved in petroleum jelly, are put on the skin under airtight dressings and examined two to four days later. The substance causing the contact dermatitis will have produced a patch of rash when the dressings are removed. A positive patch test does not, however, necessarily identify the agent causing the contact dermatitis. There must also be a history of exposure to the test agent in the areas where the dermatitis originally occurred before a definite diagnosis can be made. Extensive patch tests may have to be made to track down the offending agent. In order to minimise the number of substances tested, the patient should be questioned as to hobbies, occupation, use of cosmetics, creams and ointments, etc, to give some clues as to possible causal agents.

A huge number of substances have been implicated in causing allergic contact dermatitis. The following are some of the more common causes:

• Nickel is the most highly allergenic metal and is used in jewellery, coins and clothes fasteners. Some people can even react to nickel through a layer of cloth, and there have been cases caused by contact with nickel in coins carried in the pocket and with using metal chairs. Ear-piercing is also another source of this particular allergy. A gold-plated nickel sleeper earring can cause sensitivity, and although the initial rash is confined to the ear lobe, the entire skin then becomes allergic to nickel. Stainless steel contains 5 per cent nickel, so a very large number of household fittings can affect sensitive individuals, e.g. scissors. The source of nickel allergy is easy to identify from the site of contact dermatitis. For example, a rash on the neck and chest may be caused by a necklace, at the waistline by buckles, zips and stud fastenings on jeans and skirts, and on the hands by taps, scissors, rings, thimbles or handles.

- topical drugs – many ingredients in topical drugs can constitute a major cause of allergic contact dermatitis, for example antibiotics (penicillin, sulphonamides, neomycin), antihistamines (dephenhydramine, promethazine), anaesthetics (benzocaine), antiseptics (hexachlorophene), and stabilisers used in preparations (ethylenediamine and its derivatives).
- shampoos, hair sprays and dyes, cosmetics and deodorants
- plants, including ragweed and primrose and, in the United States, poison ivy and poison oak.
- many chemicals used in the manufacture of shoes and clothing. These include tanning agents in shoes; free formaldehyde in durable-press finishes; rubber accelerators and antioxidants in gloves, shoes, underwear and other clothing.
- artificial rubber such as latex is a potent cause of con-

tact dermatitis. It is found in gloves, sponges, sticking plaster, shoes and even elastic.
- cement is a common cause of allergic contact dermatitis among bricklayers.
- lanolin (sheep's wool fat)

Photoallergic and phototoxic contact dermatitis

These particular forms of contact dermatitis require exposure to light after contact with certain substances that sensitise the skin. Agents commonly responsible for photoallergic contact dermatitis include aftershave lotions, sunscreens and some antibiotics. These agents react with substances in the skin, which trigger an allergic reaction when exposed to sunlight.

Phototoxic contact dermatitis acts in a slightly different way by concentrating ultraviolet light from the sun in the skin and causing more rapid burning. Agents responsible for this condition include perfumes, coal tar, psoralens and oils used in manufacturing processes.

Treatment for contact dermatitis

Unless the offending agent can be avoided, treatment may be ineffective or the dermatitis may promptly recur. Avoidance of some sources of the contactant is quite straightforward; for example, it is easy to stop wearing nickel jewellery. However, other contactants are quite widespread and may be more difficult to avoid. Wearing of rubber gloves when washing up or carrying out other activities involving water, detergents or solvents may help. Patients with photoallergic contact dermatitis may also have to avoid exposure to light.

For those where the source of the allergen is at work, transfer to another department may be possible, or wearing protective clothing or gloves may solve the problem. After a serious outbreak, a patient should not return to work before the condition clears up.

Treatments such as those used for eczema can be used, for example emollients and steroid creams and ointments. Oral steroids can be used in very severe or extensive cases.

Antihistamines, except for their sedative effect, and allergen desensitisation are ineffective in contact dermatitis.

6

Urticaria and Angioedema

Urticaria

Urticaria is a very common allergic skin condition. It is more commonly known as *hives* or *nettle rash*, which it resembles. About 1 in 5 people is estimated to suffer from this condition at some time in his or her life.

Urticaria is recognised by a characteristic blistering of the skin. These raised areas or bumps, referred to as *weals*, are pale in the middle and become red around the edge. The weals and the skin surrounding them become intensely itchy. This condition affects only the superficial areas of the skin. The weals typically occur in small groups anywhere on the body or they may cover a larger area of skin. They are usually quite small, 1 to 5 mm, but in a few cases they may become much larger and reach a size of up to 20 mm. These larger weals tend to clear from the centre and may be noticed first as large red rings. An urticarial rash usually lasts only a few hours and seldom for longer than 24 to 48 hours. Urticaria can come on suddenly, following an exposure to something that triggers it off, or recur in attacks lasting for months or even years without any apparent cause. Recurrent attacks lasting less than one month are regarded as acute but outbreaks that persist for longer are looked on as chronic conditions.

Causes of urticaria

There are many causes of urticaria. Some of these causes are allergic in nature, but there are also many non-allergic causes. Often the cause of urticaria is unknown, especially in chronic cases which last for more than three weeks. It is exceptional to find a specific cause for this type of urticaria, and the antibody IgE is rarely involved, indicating that this is not a typical Type I allergic reaction. Occasionally, chronic ingestion of an unsuspected drug or chemical is responsible, e.g. from penicillin that has been given to cows and gets into their milk; from the use of non-prescription drugs; or from preservatives, dyes or other food additives.

Causes of acute urticaria include:

- drug allergy, particularly to aspirin and antibiotics such as penicillin
- insect stings or bites
- pollens
- plants (nettles and strawberry leaves)
- animals
- house dust mites
- inhaled moulds – particularly when cutting grass
- parasites, such as worms – mainly in tropical countries

108

- certain foods – particularly eggs, shellfish (such as crab, prawns and lobsters) nuts (peanuts, cashews and hazelnuts) or berry fruits, especially strawberries

Some reactions occur explosively following ingestion of minute amounts of food. On the other hand, reactions to strawberries may occur only after eating large amounts of the fruit. Strawberries contain substances that cause the release of histamine from mast cells by a mechanism that does not involve allergy. Some other foods, such as old cheese and tuna fish, contain very large amounts of histamine, which, when eaten, causes the rash directly. Highly sensitive people can even react to odours from food as it is being cooked. Typical examples of such foods are fish and eggs.

Urticaria is more common in people with other allergies. About 20 per cent of hay-fever sufferers have urticaria, and it is also quite common in people with allergic eczema.

Some types of urticaria can be brought on by very different causes. One form, known as *dermatographism*, occurs in people with very sensitive skins. In this type of urticaria, a typical weal with flare appears where the skin has been stroked firmly or where the skin has been scratched without breaking the surface. In these cases, the urticarial rash is the same shape as the original scratch or follows the pattern of stroking.

Other non-allergic causes of urticaria are changes in temperature, either when a person gets too hot or too cold, infection, especially if this is accompanied by a temperature, emotion such as fear and excitement, and exposure to ultraviolet light.

What happens in an attack of urticaria?

Whatever the cause of urticaria, the blood vessel capillaries in the affected skin become leaky so that there is an outpouring of fluid into the tissue just below the skin surface. This makes the area of skin swell up. The blood supply to the affected area is increased, and so the skin becomes red and inflamed. These changes are caused by the mediators of inflammation, such as histamine from mast cells in the skin, which also give rise to the itching. Mast cells can be triggered by allergens if they are coated in IgE antibody, accounting for the allergic type of urticaria. However, mast cells can also be triggered in other ways without involving the antibody, and it is probably this mechanism that is responsible for the non-allergic attacks of urticaria.

Treatment

If the cause of urticaria is known, steps can be taken to avoid it, e.g. avoidance of particular foods. This is relatively easy in the case of acute urticaria where the reaction is so prompt and unequivocal that the food or other agent causing the condition can be easily identified. In chronic urticaria, where the cause of the rash is, more often than not, unknown, this is more difficult. Only about 20 to 30 per cent of people with chronic urticaria ever find out what causes their condition.

Acute urticaria is a self-limiting condition that generally subsides in one to seven days. Many people do not require any treatment at all but oral, non-sedative antihistamines can be taken to relieve symptoms if necessary. All non-essential drugs should be stopped until the reaction has subsided. If the urticaria does not settle rapidly, a diet low in azo dyes, preservatives and colourings should be taken as one of these may be the cause of the condition. If the urticaria persists, a short course of a steroid such as predisolone may be necessary for one or two weeks.

In approximately half the cases of chronic urticaria, the condition clears itself within about two years. The control of stress often helps reduce the frequency and severity of the episodes. Coffee, alcohol, tobacco smoking and certain drugs, e.g. aspirin, may aggravate symptoms and so these should be avoided. Oral histamines with a tranquillising effect are usually beneficial. A diet low in histamine may be worth trying in cases of chronic urticaria. The foods to be avoided are well-ripened cheeses, continental sausages and tinned fish, such as tuna and mackerel, which can contain high levels of histamine.

Some of the naturally occurring bacteria in the gut produce histamine. If the diet is high in vegetables, fruit and starchy foods, then the levels of histamine produced may be excessive. If urticaria gets worse after eating a

meal then it is possible that bacterial-produced histamine is the cause of the condition. A diet low in fruit,
vegetables and starch could be tried to see if the condition improves. Inclusion of live yoghurt in the diet may
also help to improve the balance of bacteria in the gut.

Angioedema

Angioedema is a rare condition that is similar to urticaria but the swelling is usually more extensive. This condition involves the deeper layers of skin and the underlying subcutaneous tissues. Unlike urticaria, angioedema is not itchy but it can be painful or cause a burning
sensation. About 50 per cent of people who suffer from
urticaria also suffer from angioedema. However, some
people get angioedema but not urticaria.

All areas of the body can be affected, and in some
cases widespread swelling of the face, eyes, mouth, lips
and throat occurs. Gross distortion of the face may occur in severe cases, the eyes becoming swollen to mere
slits and the lips grotesquely enlarged. The limbs, particularly the joints, may also be involved and become so
swollen that they are difficult to bend. When the digestive system is affected, the internal swelling can cause
severe abdominal pain. In very rare cases the condition
can become life-threatening when the vocal cords,
throat and other parts of the airways become swollen,
presenting problems with breathing. In these cases,
medical attention should be sought immediately and

adrenaline can be given to relieve the condition. If medical help is delayed for any reason then it may be that the only resort is to insert a breathing tube into the trachea to administer oxygen in this way. A Medic-alert pendant or bracelet is often worn by people who suffer from this severe condition so that appropriate help can be given promptly if necessary. Some individuals, under a doctor's advice, also carry adrenaline to administer to themselves if the need arises. The adrenaline is carried in a syringe to make self-administration easier, and these individuals are taught to give themselves subcutaneous or intramuscular injections. In less severe cases, antihistamine drugs can be given.

As in urticaria, the swelling is probably the result of the action of mast cells in the lower layers of the skin. When these cells degranulate, they release mediators that cause the blood capillaries serving the tissues to become leaky. Serum, the watery part of the blood, then seeps into the tissues, causing the characteristic swelling. In angioedema this leaking of serum into the tissues is more marked.

Angioedema can be caused by allergies, but there are also many other causes of the condition. It can also be symptomatic of a number of serious, underlying disorders, and these should be investigated and eliminated before the possible role of allergy is examined.

Many of the allergic causes of urticaria also cause angioedema. However, inahalants such as pollens and house dust mites are less likely to cause the condition (*see* Urticaria). Drugs such as aspirin are a more common cause of this condition than of urticaria. In people who already have some underlying allergic condition, sunshine, excessive temperatures and emotional stress can all trigger the symptoms of angioedema.

Hereditary angioedema

This form of angioedema is not allergic in nature but is an hereditary condition. It is the result of a lack of a particular enzyme in the blood. Angioedema attacks associated with this condition usually occur regularly and are rarely associated with urticaria. Prolonged treatment with hormones or drugs that affect blood clotting is required.

7

Food Allergies

Allergies to food are the least well understood and perhaps the most controversial. It is also the area of allergy in which the descriptive terms are not used consistently – which adds to the confusion.

A number of claims for food allergy are controversial – for example, that allergy to food or food additives can be responsible for hyperactivity in children or the 'tension-fatigue syndrome'. There are also claims that food allergy is to blame for a range of conditions such as arthritis, obesity and depression. There is little evidence to substantiate these claims. However, it is quite possible that some *may* be implicated, although with the current level of knowledge it is not clear which foods are involved or exactly how.

The food we eat may have a wide range of ill-effects on the body, which can bring about a variety of symptoms. These effects have a range of causes including:

- contamination of food by bacteria and other infectious organisms
- a true allergy to food in which the immune system and IgE antibodies are involved

- food intolerance, which may be the result of, among other things, an enzyme deficiency or a sensitivity to particular chemicals in various foods
- a toxic-like effect of high levels of histamine in certain foods
- immunological disease, where antibodies other than IgE antibodies are involved, e.g. in coeliac disease (*see* section on coeliac disease later in chapter).

Every day we take in a wide range of foods that may contain additives for preserving purposes or to enhance flavour and colour. Yeasts and fungi may also be found in foodstuffs, especially in grains. Because of the wide variety of foods eaten, it might be supposed that allergies to them would be more common. However, the body has a variety of mechanisms that protect it from the large amount of potential allergens in the diet while absorbing necessary nutrients. The body's immune defences are able to discriminate between essential food substances and potentially harmful organisms and toxins, and this process is employed in defending the gastrointestinal system. The prevention of gastrointestinal infection depends largely on the local defences of the mucous surfaces of the lining of the digestive tract.

The presence of particular antibodies – immunoglobulin A (IgA) in the lining of the gut can react with foreign proteins, rendering them non-allergic. The body can sometimes adapt and tolerate allergens to which it is continually exposed.

The cooking of foods and the natural processes of digestion can reduce the potency of many food allergens. The effectiveness of digestion in preventing food allergy symptoms in most adults is considerable. Many allergic individuals will react to an inhaled allergen, or on contact, but not when they eat the substance. One example of this is in the condition known as baker's asthma. Affected workers wheeze on exposure to flour dust and show positive skin tests to wheat and/or other grains. However, they suffer no adverse effects when they eat grain products.

In some instances, people do not react to food every time they eat it. For example, they may find that they can eat chicken that has been fed on one type of grain with no ill effects but may react on another occasion. In this case, the person is probably reacting to a component of the food that was fed to the chickens rather than to the chicken meat itself.

The term *food allergy* is used very loosely and is sometimes incorrectly applied to many adverse reactions to food that are not strictly allergy. The term food allergy should only be used to mean those adverse reactions to food that involve the immune system and primarily the production of IgE antibodies in response to a food allergen. The definitions of terms applied to the reactions to food, such as 'food sensitivity' and 'food intolerance', also vary considerably. The terms as they are used in this chapter are defined below.

Food aversion

Food aversion is a purely psychological response to a food, which results in a person disliking or avoiding a particular food. It may be that they have had a bad experience with the food previously if, say, it was contaminated and caused food poisoning, and so never want it again. There is no physical reason why they should avoid the food.

Food allergy

Food allergy can be defined as an adverse reaction to a food in which the immune system reacts inappropriately or abnormally to a foodstuff that in most people causes no such problem. The production of IgE antibodies are involved in this response and also possibly mast cells. Typically, the allergic response develops shortly after eating and can be caused by the smallest trace of the food. There are some instances where an allergic response has occurred when a saucepan which has previously been used to cook the offending food has not been washed properly. When the saucepan is used again, the remaining traces of the food are enough to elicit an allergic response. The allergic reaction happens each time the specific food is encountered. A positive skin prick test (described in Chapter 10) is usually taken as proof that the immune system is involved. People who suffer from food allergies usually also have other allergies such as eczema or hay fever, and the condition often runs in families. Using this definition, fewer than 1 per cent of adults and 5 per cent of children suffer from true food allergies, and they are certainly far less common than is generally believed.

Many foods have been reported as causing allergy. Milk, eggs, fish (particularly shellfish) and nuts (particularly peanuts) are the most important.

When food allergy is severe, the first mouthful can cause dramatic swelling of the lips, tongue and throat. In some cases this can be life-threatening if the swelling of the mouth and throat prevents breathing. Occasionally, sufficient food allergen is absorbed into the bloodstream to cause a widespread allergic response, called anaphylaxis, in which the development of severe asthma is combined with a rapid fall in blood pressure. Death can ensue if medical help is not obtained immediately. Anaphylaxis may also occur in people who do not usually react so violently if they take exercise after eating the food in question.

Less severe allergy causes typical symptoms in the digestive system, especially colic and diarrhoea. Sometimes food allergy can also cause asthma and nasal symptoms.

False food allergies some food allergies are caused by foods triggering mast cells directly. These allergies are sometimes referred to as false food allergies because they do not involve the immune system and do not depend on IgE antibodies being formed. The end result of this process is exactly similar to an allergic response and the symptoms are indistinguishable. Foods that can act in this way include tomatoes, strawberries, chocolate, shellfish, pork and alcohol.

Food intolerance

Food intolerance is used here as an umbrella term for all those adverse food reactions that do not include either a psychological rejection of food (food aversion) or a largely immune response to food (food allergy). Food intolerance can be defined as an adverse reaction to a specific food where negative skin prick tests and other tests for allergy suggest there is no involvement of the immune system. This does not necessarily exclude all involvement of the immune system but it is not primarily implicated. Intolerance covers a wide range of responses, including those caused by a lack of vital enzymes for the digestion of a particular food and certain food sensitivities.

Unlike allergy, the reactions involved in food intolerance are not immediate and usually build up over time. Larger amounts of the food are needed to provoke symptoms, unlike food allergy, where very minute traces are sufficient. The reaction is often to some food that is eaten regularly, such as wheat or milk, and as the symptoms are quite mild at first it is often difficult to diagnose the problem. For these reasons, at one time these conditions were referred to as 'masked' or 'delayed' food allergies. The symptoms of food intolerance can disappear altogether if the food is excluded from the diet for a few months and may be tolerated at a future date if the food is eaten occasionally in small quantities.

Unlike food allergy, there are no typical symptoms and probably no single mechanism involved. Food intolerance is a complex subject and few generalisations can be made.

It is often difficult to say when the condition started as there is a gradual onset of symptoms that slowly get worse. The number of symptoms may also gradually accumulate over time, and individuals may become intolerant of more and more foods. Occasionally, a severe case of influenza or diarrhoea may set off a case of food intolerance.

There is a wide variation in the symptoms associated with food intolerance, and most systems within the body may be affected. As might be expected, many of these symptoms affect some part of the gastro-intestinal system but others, such as migraine, depression, fatigue and water retention (oedema), are also common. (See Table 7.1 for some of the symptoms associated with food intolerance). Some conditions are discussed more fully later in the chapter.

As if to emphasise the complex nature of food intolerance, symptoms associated with it often come and go or vary in their severity. It is thought that this may bebecause of factors other than food which may exacerbate symptoms. These factors may include stress levels or

> **Table 7.1: Some symptoms and conditions caused or contributed to by food intolerance**
>
> - Rheumatoid arthritis
> - Migraine
> - Asthma
> - Infantile colic
> - Mouth ulcers
> - Urticaria
> - Eczema and other skin rashes
> - Angioedema
> - Depression
> - Crohn's disease and ulcerative colitis
> - Fatigue and excessive sleepiness
> - Coeliac disease
> - Irritable bowel syndrome (constipation and/or diarrhoea, bloating, abdominal pain, wind)

hormone fluctuations, e.g. in the menstrual cycle. Specific foods do not necessarily cause the same symptoms in everyone.

The foods involved in intolerance are varied, but those most often associated with it include:

- wheat, rye, oats, maize
- milk and milk products
- beef
- hen's eggs and chicken meat

- tea, coffee
- chocolate
- sugar
- colourings and preservatives
- yeast
- pork
- peanuts
- citrus fruits
- alcohol

Enzyme deficiency one particular type of intolerance may be the result of the body being unable to handle the food because of a lack of an enzyme that is important in its digestion prior to absorption. The commonest example of this is absence of lactase, the enzyme needed to break down the sugar in milk. Some people cannot digest milk and milk products properly because of low levels of this enzyme. Whenever they take these foods they suffer from crampy abdominal pain and diarrhoea. Some children are born without the enzyme and develop severe watery diarrhoea when fed with milk. If the condition goes unrecognised, the child fails to thrive, and collapse and death can follow. As the child grows older, milk does not play such an important part in the diet. In races where milk is not common in the diet, for example in the Chinese, levels of lactase are very low and drinking milk leads to diarrhoea. Levels of lactase can also be reduced by many common bowel disorders, such as gastro-enteritis, and drinking milk can lead to diarrhoea for many months following the illness. Similarly, many Asians feel ill after drinking even small amounts of alcohol because they lack the enzyme that breaks down its by-products. Neither of these conditions occurs if only small amounts of the food are consumed.

Food sensitivity is another type of food intolerance. Some people find that an existing medical condition can be triggered or exacerbated after eating a particular food. This is known as a food sensitivity. Chemicals that affect blood vessels are found in many foods. High concentrations of one such chemical, tyramine, is present in some cheeses and pickled fish. A similar chemical, called phenylethylamine, is found in chocolate, and citrus fruits contain octoamine. These and similar compounds occur in bananas, avocado, yeast extract and wine. A person who suffers from migraine often finds these foods bring on such attacks.

Conditions and symptoms associated with food intolerance and food allergy

Many conditions associated with food allergy and food intolerance are not well understood, and neither are the mechanisms and the role played by diet. Many conditions are probably not caused only by allergy or intolerance but a combination of both, as will become clear in the following section.

Migraine

Headaches are a very common condition, and many of the population suffer from them from time to time. Recurrent headaches are often reported as a feature of food intolerance. Migraine is a particularly severe headache often affecting just one side of the head. It is often accompanied by nausea and vomiting. Some sufferers also experience visual disturbance, such as flashing lights and split vision; in addition, bright lights and loud noise may disturb them. Most people experience their first migraine between the ages of 20 and 50, but in some, migraines first develop in childhood. It is estimated that about 1 in 10 of the population suffers from this condition, and more women are affected than men.

Many patients recognise that various things can trigger their migraines, e.g. fatigue, loud noises, anxiety, stress, changes in climate, high winds and premenstrual tension. Some sufferers report that migraines occur after eating certain foods. The most commonly implicated foods are chocolate, cheese and, in some cases, alcohol, particularly red wine. Current thinking suggests that true allergy is not involved in the development of migraines – it is thought more likely to be a sensitivity to certain chemicals found in food. The chemicals implicated in this condition are amines, and in particular two types – tyramine and phenylamine. Both these can cause blood vessels to dilate. It is believed that it is the expansion of the blood vessels in the brain that causes the pain associated with migraine. There is some evidence that migraine sufferers do not produce enough of the enzymes needed to break down the chemicals. High concentrations of amines are found in some cheeses, chocolate and red wine. Other examples of amine-containing foods are beef, yeast extract, broad beans, pineapple, banana and avocado.

Most migraine attacks can be treated with simple analgesics, such as paracetamol, to alleviate the symptoms. However, if a particular trigger can be identified then steps can be taken to avoid it and so prevent the onset of an attack. If migraines are particularly severe then drugs that act on the blood vessels may be advised.

Arthritis

Arthritis is a general term for painful swelling and stiffness of the joints, and there are many different forms caused by a variety of factors. Arthritis can accompany or follow all sorts of diseases, such as influenza, rheumatic fever, German measles and Salmonella infection. Food intolerance is also reported as bringing on joint pain. It has been known for a long time that one form of the disease, gout, can be brought on by eating certain foods. Studies have shown that some patients respond well to elimination diets, indicating that food intolerance may be involved in at least some cases of arthritis.

It is suspected that the pain in arthritis is caused by complexes being formed in the blood and then being deposited in the joints. These complexes consist of a mixture of antibodies and antigens. Where this condition is thought to be brought on by food intolerance, a similar mechanism could be at work. In this case, the immune complexes would probably consist of food molecules and antibodies to them. There is no actual evidence that this is the mechanism at work but it is one possibility, although there may well be others.

Rheumatoid arthritis is a common chronic and disabling form of arthritis. It is characterised by painful, swollen joints that feel warm to the touch and are often stiff. The stiffness and pain are usually worse in the morning. Initially, it is inflammation of the synovial membrane that causes the stiffness, as this membrane produces a fluid that lubricates the joint. The inflammation then spreads to other parts of the joint. The cause of the condition is unknown, but the immune system is involved, as is indicated by the large numbers of immune cells that surround the synovial membrane in affected patients. It is these cells that are responsible for causing the inflammation.

It was the presence of the immune cells in the joints that suggested that rheumatoid arthritis might involve a bacterial or viral infection, but no organism has ever been found despite years of research. This explanation now seems unlikely. A more recent theory is that rheumatoid arthritis is, in fact, an autoimmune disease and that the body is mounting an immune reaction against its own proteins.

Food intolerance may have a part to play in this form of arthritis but, as yet, there is no strong evidence for this. The condition does show improvement in some patients who go on an elimination diet, and occasionally there is a dramatic improvement and patients may become free of symptoms altogether.

Hyperactivity

Hyperactive children are impulsive and excitable. They usually have poor concentration and are difficult to control. They often require little sleep and/or experience disturbed sleep patterns. There is also a tendency for them to have temper tantrums. Although these children have normal IQs, they often have learning difficulties and do not do well at school. Some hyperactive children can also display hostile and aggressive behaviour but this is not always the case. Other hyperactive children are happy individuals.

The causes of hyperactivity are not known, but food allergy and food intolerance appear to play a part in the condition in at least some cases. One study carried out in Canada found that 20 per cent of cases could be attributed to a food allergy in which IgE antibodies were involved. Most hyperactive children also display other allergic conditions such as eczema, urticaria, migraine and diarrhoea. They are also usually sensitive to pollens, house dust, household chemicals and some food additives. Elimination diets have produced improvements in the condition of many children. Use of these diets has found that hyperactive children may be sensitive to naturally occurring salicylates (aspirin-like compounds) that are found in fruits and vegetables as well as in certain food additives. However, in most of these cases, other common allergens such as pollens and house dust were also important. Improvements in the condition could be achieved in a majority of cases when most of these allergens were excluded.

One theory put forward for the action of food additives in hyperactivity is that affected children may be lacking in, or have low levels of, the necessary enzyme to break down the chemical compounds. More work is needed to investigate this and to determine the importance of diet for hyperactive children.

Coeliac disease

Coeliac disease is a disorder of the small intestine caused by an intolerance to the protein gluten. This protein is found in cereals such as wheat, rye and, to a lesser extent, in barley and oats. Its name derives from the Greek word *koiliakos*, 'belly'. The condition is also known as gluten enteropathy – enteropathy meaning disease of the bowel.

Coeliac disease was first recognised in the Second World War when it was noticed that the condition of sickly children who suffered from persistent diarrhoea improved when they were on the restricted wartime diet that included very little bread. It is now known that glia-din, a protein found in gluten, acts as an antigen and combines with antibodies to form an immune complex in the lining of the intestine. This complex attracts K (killer) lymphocytes. In some way, which is not entirely clear, the complex severely damages the lining of the digestive system so that absorption of nutrients and wa-ter from food is severely reduced. This results in typical watery diarrhoea, and children suffering from the dis-ease are thin and weak and often anaemic.

Coeliac disease is not often thought of as food intoler-ance but it is an adverse reaction to food. Although it is not a true allergic condition, as defined in this text, since it does not involve IgE antibodies, the immune system is nonetheless involved. IgG and IgA antibodies are found in the bloodstream of many people who suffer from the disease.

The tendency to develop coeliac disease is inherited and often runs in families. Family members are also likely to suffer from other allergic conditions. Severe cases of coeliac disease often become apparent in infan-cy. Less severe cases, which may have fewer specific symptoms, may go undetected for many years. Coeliac disease in babies does not become apparent until a few weeks after they are weaned. Prior to being diagnosed, the infant fails to thrive and produces pale, foul-smell-ing stools. Other symptoms include wind and bloating and, in some cases, the child becomes anaemic. When the condition begins in adulthood, symptoms include diarrhoea, pain, bloating, weight loss, malaise and weakness. In contrast, the only symptom in some people is constipation.

If coeliac disease is suspected then it can be confirmed with a bowel biopsy (a small sample of tissue), which reveals damage to the lining of the bowel. If the biopsy is positive, then the only treatment is the complete avoidance of gluten. Complete avoidance can be difficult to achieve because cereals containing gluten are widely used in commercial soups, sauces, ice creams, sausages, etc. In order to avoid foods containing gluten, people with this condition need detailed lists of foodstuffs and their constituents. Some of the large food manufacturers now label many of their gluten-free products to aid the consumer.

In most cases, coeliac disease is a lifelong condition. The only exception to this is in the case of a few infants in whom, if the condition is diagnosed early enough, the condition may be reversible. While most coeliacs have to avoid all traces of gluten, some are able to tolerate small amounts occasionally and some can eat oats, which contain lower levels. However, it is risky for patients to experiment with gluten as some have an acute reaction to even a small amount. This is known as *coeliac shock*.

A few patients respond poorly to the withdrawal of gluten from the diet. This may be because of an incorrect diagnosis or because the lining of the gut is so badly damaged that it may take some time to repair itself. Zinc supplements are sometimes given to aid this process. In some cases an individual may be intolerant to other foods as well as gluten. This may have been precipitated by damage to the gut as a result of coeliac disease. An additional intolerance to soya may often develop as it is widely used in gluten-free products. Intolerances to milk, fish, rice and chicken also occur. An elimination diet can be tried to track down the offending foodstuff.

Irritable bowel syndrome (IBS)

This is a common condition, and it is estimated that approximately half of all people complaining of gastro-intestinal problems suffer from irritable bowel syndrome. About three times as many women suffer from this condition as men.

This condition, also known as *irritable colon* or *spastic colon*, comprises an abnormal function of the bowel. The main symptoms are attacks of diarrhoea and abdominal pain alternating with episodes of constipation, although some patients suffer from diarrhoea most of the time while others are often constipated. Most also suffer pain that is relieved after defecation. There may also be belching, flatulence, abdominal bloating and distension. A number of diseases can produce the same symptoms, but in irritable bowel syndrome there is no sign of infection or other physical damage, including bowel cancer or an ulcer. The general health of the patients with irritable bowel syndrome is not altered, and there is usually no weight loss. In most cases, the condition does not get worse with time.

It is not clear whether the condition is caused by food allergy, food intolerance or neither. Other suggestions for its cause are that it is psychosomatic in origin, or the result of a lack of fibre in the diet. However, some studies have shown that as many as 70 per cent of sufferers may be food intolerant.

A number of people with this condition find that it is triggered by various foods and that the condition improves if they avoid the offending substances. Foods commonly associated with IBS are cereals, milk, dairy products, eggs, chocolate, coffee, tea, nuts, citrus fruit, some spices and certain vegetables. Irritant foods such as hot, spicy dishes can also exacerbate the condition.

It is thought that irritable bowel syndrome may be caused by spasm of the smooth muscle in the bowel, but what brings this about is unclear. If the condition is indeed a food allergy, it may be that mast cells are responsible. Another theory is that the condition is the result of an imbalance in the flora (bacteria and yeasts) that inhabit the gut. There may be too many of some kinds but too few of others, and these may be responsible for the symptoms.

Crohn's disease

Crohn's disease is severe inflammation of the lower part of the small intestine (the ileum) or the large intestine (the colon). It is a serious disease and can obstruct the passage of food through the gut. Patients with this disease suffer from cramps, generalised abdominal pain and diarrhoea.

The patches of inflammation in this condition have a characteristic appearance under the microscope. In some cases, the inflammation may heal itself, and some patients experience only one or two episodes of the disease. In others the disease may recur again and again.

Victims of Crohn's disease may suffer generalised abdominal pain, especially after eating, and there is a feeling of malaise and sometimes a slight fever. If the condition continues untreated, weight loss and general ill-health follow. Other common symptoms are mouth ulcers and joint pain.

The cause of the disease is unknown but food intolerance seems to be implicated. Studies have shown that many individuals can recover when put on elimination diets but react again when a specific food is reintroduced. As Crohn's disease is a serious condition, elimination diets should be undertaken only with medical supervision. Often the patient is initially put on an elemental diet, which contains all the necessary nutrients but in a broken-down form, before going on to a proper elimination diet. Whether these diets work by resting the bowel, changing the bacterial content or reducing allergy is not certain.

Conventional treatment for Crohn's disease is to use corticosteroids to suppress the inflammation. If scarring in the bowel is severe and causing congestion then surgery may be needed.

Ulcerative colitis

Ulcerative colitis is another inflammatory disease of the large intestine (the colon). Symptoms include episodes of severe abdominal pain and diarrhoea that is often bloody and contains mucus. Tiredness, weakness and lack of energy are also common among patients with this condition. At one time it was thought that ulcerative colitis was related to milk intolerance, but this now seems unlikely, as when patients are put on elemental diets or fed intravenously there is no sustained improvement in their condition. Although ulcerative colitis can afflict patients of any age, it is more likely to affect people aged 15 to 30 years. There is also a small peak in the number of people suffering the condition later in life, particularly between the ages of 50 to 70. As with Crohn's disease, the cause is not clear and food intolerance is just one possibility.

Another form that is commonly caused by food is infant colitis, especially in a baby under one year old. This is a rare condition, and the main symptom is diarrhoea containing blood and mucus. It is thought that food intolerance is a factor in about 75 per cent of cases. There are clear signs that the immune system is involved, and in some babies, IgE antibodies and mast cells are found. In other cases it is believed that another type of immune reaction is involved. Infant colitis can therefore be a true food allergy, and in these cases the condition is known as *food-allergic colitis*. Most affected babies are bottle-fed, but occasionally the baby is breast-fed and is reacting to some food the mother is eating that is passing to the baby. In the case of bottle-fed babies, the condition can be remedied by switching to a hydrolysate formula based on milk but in which the proteins are partially broken down so it is not so likely to provoke allergy. When the baby is breast-fed, the mother simply has to eliminate the food from her diet. The most common foods implicated are milk, soya, egg and wheat.

Food allergy and children

The tendency to develop allergies is often an inherited characteristic and can therefore run in families. However, a family history does not mean that that particular child will develop allergies. A number of steps can be taken to reduce the chances of a child developing allergies to food or food intolerance.

Food allergy appears to be less likely in babies who are breast-fed, and certain foods should be introduced into the diet later rather than sooner. These include all those foodstuffs most commonly associated with allergic conditions, such as cow's milk, eggs, peanuts, fish, wheat and other cereals containing gluten. Guidelines issued by the Department of Health suggest babies should be breast-fed or bottle-fed until they are at least four months old. Other foods can then be introduced as follows:

4–6 months old	vegetables, fruit (other than citrus fruits), rice, meat, chicken, and pulses (e.g. lentils)
6–12 months old	foods containing wheat (e.g. pasta, bread, biscuits), fish, eggs, yoghurt, cheese and citrus fruits
over 12 months old	ordinary cow's milk

It is recommended that peanuts and products containing them should not be introduced into the diet until after the child is at least 12 months old. In atopic families, in which allergies are present, they should not be introduced until after the child is five years old.

Foods implicated in food allergy or food intolerance

An allergy to one food may sometimes result in a similar allergic reaction to other closely related ones. For example, an allergy to wheat may mean a person is also allergic to other related cereals such as rye, barley or oats. This is known as *cross-reactivity*. It is thought that IgE antibodies that bind with the antigens of one food may also bind with proteins of a similar structure in a related substance. Cross-reactivity is also observed in food intolerance, but in this case the mechanism is unknown.

Cross-reactions are more common within certain groups of foods, including cereals, shellfish, fish and nuts. Cross-reactivity is also found between certain pollens and foods (*see* the section on nuts which follows). However, cross-reactivity is rare within groups of animal foodstuffs and so, for example, people who are allergic to cow's milk can often eat beef. The proteins found in milk are not similar to those found in beef.

Milk and milk products

Cow's milk is a common cause of allergy in infancy and in childhood. The allergy is controversial, as immune reactions can be demonstrated only in a small proportion of patients. As described earlier, some people suffer from an intolerance to cow's milk rather than allergy. This may be because of a lack of the enzyme lactase, which means that milk can neither be digested or absorbed.

It is almost impossible for human breast milk to cause an allergy unless the mother has been taking an allergy-producing drug or chemical that passes into the breast milk and hence to the baby. Cutting milk out of an infant's diet can have serious nutritional consequences, especially in developing countries. Goat's milk can be given as a substitute, although in some cases. an infant may also develop an allergy to this. 'Milk' made from soya beans can also be used as a substitute for cow's milk, and it is available in a number of infant formulas. After babyhood, milk can be cut out of the diet altogether as it is not essential to life, although other sources of calcium should be included in the diet.

Eggs

Eggs are an important cause of food allergy. It is the protein in egg white that is the most important source of allergen. The MMR (measles, mumps and rubella) vaccine may contain minute traces of egg protein as it is usually grown on a media containing this substance. If a child is allergic to egg white, the family doctor should be advised of this so that the vaccine can be checked to confirm that it is free of the protein. If the egg allergy is known to produce severe symptoms in the child, then a skin prick test should be used to test the vaccine before it is administered. If no response occurs, then the vaccine can be given safely. This process should be carried out in a hospital setting, in the rare event that the child may experience a reaction.

Fish

Fish, especially shellfish, can be the source of very potent allergens. In very sensitive patients, even the inhalation of steam from cooking fish can cause asthma. Some people are allergic to only one species of fish and can tolerate other types. People who are sensitive to shellfish are not necessarily sensitive to bony fish, and vice versa.

Allergic reactions to fish can cause a range of symptoms, including rashes, itching, swelling of the mouth and face, and wheezing. Reactions to some fish, especially shellfish, including shrimps, lobster and crab, can be very violent and even life-threatening. Victims of this type of reaction can suffer anaphylactic shock (*see* chapter on anaphylaxis). If a person reacts violently to one type of fish, it is probably wise to avoid all fish in the diet.

Nuts

Many different kinds of nuts cause allergic reactions in sensitive people, and sometimes these are very severe. Nuts known to cause allergic responses include walnuts, almonds, cashews, pistachio nuts, hazelnuts, pecans and peanuts (also known as groundnuts). People are often sensitive to more than one type of nut. Some nuts are closely related and are similar to each other in their chemical make-up. Hence people who are allergic to walnuts are often allergic to almonds, and in the same way allergies to cashews and pistachio nuts often go together. In some cases, however, people can be allergic to nuts that are not related and may have very different chemical compositions. Other instances of cross-reactivity between the same plant families are found; for example, people who are allergic to birch pollen also frequently react to hazelnuts.

Symptoms associated with nut allergy include swelling of the lips, mouth and tongue and the development of urticaria or nettle rash. In severe cases, the reaction can be very serious, resulting in collapse from anaphylactic shock (*see* chapter on anaphylaxis). Some people are so sensitive that even the merest trace of the nut may cause a serious response. One in every 500 adults and one in every 1000 children has an acute severe reaction to nuts each year. About one in a million of these is fatal.

Allergy to peanuts is perhaps the most well-known. In fact, the peanut is really a legume, belonging to the same plant family as peas and beans. Allergy to both peanuts and other legumes, such as peas or beans, is very unlikely. However, if an allergy to peanuts is confirmed then all nuts and products containing them should be avoided. This is because peanuts are relatively cheap and are often used as a substitute for more expensive nuts. Their flavour can be washed out and replaced with that of a different nut such as walnut or brazil. So it is wiser to avoid all nuts in food products unless the identity of the nut can be confirmed with certainty.

Peanuts are used widely in many processed foods, often in the form of vegetable oil. Under food labelling regulations, the precise source of the oil does not have to be identified and so peanut or groundnut oil will often go under the name of vegetable oil. Products containing vegetable oil should therefore be avoided by anyone with a peanut allergy. As people have become more aware of peanut allergy and its possible fatal consequences, however, many food manufacturers are beginning to label products that may contain nuts.

Nut oils can also be found in some cosmetic creams

and preparations and so care should be taken to examine the constituents of such products.

Cereals

Allergic reactions can occur as a result of products made from various cereals, including: wheat, rye, barley, oat, corn, rice. There is cross-reactivity between wheat, rye and barley, which all belong to the same family.

Soya beans

Soya bean is often used as a substitute source of protein, for example, for cow's milk. Occasionally an allergic reaction can develop.

Food additives

Additives can be defined as substances, other than nutrients, that are added intentionally to food to increase shelf life, to assist in processing and to improve palatability and appearance. There are many types of food additives, and they are classified according to the purposes for which they are used. The main groups are listed in Table 7.2.

Most additives are denoted by an 'E' prefix. Under European legislation, all foods containing additives, with the exception of flavourings, must have the E number or its name in the list of ingredients. Many additives are natural products and have been used for many

Table 7.2: The main groups of food additives and their purpose

	E numbers	Purpose of additive
Colourings	E100–E180	to make food look more attractive
Preservatives	E200–E297	to prevent bacterial growth and give the product longer shelf life
Flavourings	No E–number required	to improve flavour that is often lost in processing
Antioxidants	E300–E321	to prevent action of oxygen on food, e.g. stop fruit going brown when exposed to air
Emulsifiers and stabilisers	E322–E495	to improve the texture of the food
Flavour enhancers	E620–E635	to enhance flavour of foods

years, e.g. salt. More recently, numerous additives have been developed to perform all sorts of functions in food products. Even though an additive has an 'E' prefix, denoting that it is regarded as safe by the European Union, it does not mean that it cannot provoke an adverse reaction when eaten by some people.

Despite the wide range of additives added to food, very few have been positively linked to allergies or food intolerance. The groups of additives most often linked to producing symptoms are colourings and preservatives. In the first group interest has centred on:

- *Tartrazine (E102)* – a yellow dye found in many sweets and soft drinks, known to bring on asthma attacks and suspected of provoking hyperactivity.
- *Amaranth (E123)* – an azo dye, also suspected of being implicated in provoking asthma and hyperactivity.

Among the preservatives attention has mainly focused on:

- *Sodium bisulphite (E222)* – an antioxidant widely used in helping to keep fruit and vegetables looking fresh in salad bars, etc. It is also found in canned and dried foods, soft drinks and wine, packet sauces, soup and gravy mixes. It is believed to cause asthma.

Other preservatives, such as the benzoates (E210–E219), are suspected of causing asthma and allergic skin reactions such as urticaria, while potassium nitrate (E252) may cause skin problems and hyperactivity.

Most reactions to food additives are believed to be very rare, but it is advisable for people with asthma to avoid tartrazine and sodium bisulphate. Both these should be clearly marked on food labels.

Not only newer artificial additives have been implicated in allergy. Recently, three cases of severe allergic
reaction, anaphylaxis, have been reported in the United
States, caused by cochineal. This is a red food colouring
extracted from the cochineal beetle and has been in use
for many years. In one of the three cases, a woman had
eaten an ice lolly that had been coloured with cochineal
and this caused the anaphylactic reaction.

Foods that rarely cause allergies

There are some foods that rarely, if ever, cause food allergies, and these often form the basis of elimination diets. They include a variety of fruit and vegetables: ap-
ples, pears, grapes, peaches, plums, carrots, potatoes,
rice, green beans, marrows and courgettes. Turkey and
lamb are rarely implicated in food allergies. Amongst
the grains, only barley, oats and rye can be recommended as non-allergic, although they do contain gluten and
so must be avoided if a patient suffers from coeliac disease (*see* section on coeliac disease in this chapter).

Histamine in food

Some foods contain large amounts of histamine and,
when eaten, they can have an adverse effect on the body.
Histamines are the main chemicals produced by mast
cells to provoke an allergic reaction and so the eating of
foods rich in histamines may result in similar effects.

Histamine is formed in foods by the action of certain

bacteria. Well-ripened cheeses and continental-type sausages, especially if they are kept for a long time, are two foods that often contain high levels. High levels of histamine are found in some fish, such as mackerel and tuna, particularly if they are not kept at a low enough temperature before being eaten or canned. Some alcoholic drinks are also rich in histamines.

The main symptoms of excess levels of histamine are nausea, diarrhoea, skin rashes, flushing and headaches. These symptoms are usually short-lived as the liver is well equipped to break down histamines. Some people with pre-existing medical conditions such as cirrhosis of the liver, viral hepatitis and chronic urticaria may be more susceptible to the action of histamine, as are those taking certain drugs, such as isoniazid which is used in the treatment of tuberculosis. In the latter case the liver's ability to break down histamine is reduced.

Eating foods rich in histamine should not be confused with false-food allergy. In the former, histamines are taken into the body within the food and provoke reactions as described above. In the case of false-food allergy, the food itself acts on the mast cells within the body to release histamine. Although the effects might be the same the mechanism is different.

Elimination diets

The cause of a severe food allergy is usually obvious to the patient. However, when the reaction is not so severe or symptoms do not appear until several hours after eating, pinpointing the food that is responsible can be difficult. This may be further complicated if the patient is reacting to several foods.

Elimination diets are a way of determining the relationship between foods and symptoms. Foods suspected of causing the symptoms are removed from the diet to see if the condition improves. If it does improve, the offending foodstuff is then reintroduced into the diet to determine whether it is capable of inducing the symptoms. When a food is reintroduced, known as a *positive challenge*, it is done in a such a way that it is not recognised by the patient or the person administering the diet. This ensures that any prejudice in the outcome of the results is removed. The positive challenge can be given in the form of a capsule containing an extract of the food suspected of producing symptoms.

The basic elimination diet can be one in which the food suspected of causing symptoms is removed or the patient is put on a diet composed only of foods that are known to be relatively non-allergenic. The foods most commonly incriminated in food allergy, such as milk, eggs, shellfish, nuts, wheat, peanuts and chocolate or any products containing them, as well as particular suspected foods, should be removed from the basic diet. No other foods or fluids should be taken while on the diet, and care must be taken to ensure that all products are pure and free from other substances.

A common elimination diet consists of pears, turkey

and rice. In the United States, the turkey is often replaced by lamb as this is less frequently eaten there and so fewer people are sensitised to it. This is quite a severe diet and would be necessary only if a person were suspected of being allergic to several foods. Other diets include a greater variety of vegetables, particularly those that are not eaten very often or in any quantity, such as parsnips, turnips or carrots.

Whichever diet is chosen, if improvement is not noted within a week then another diet should be tried. If symptoms are relieved, one new food can be reintroduced into the diet at a time, about a week apart, to discover which produces symptoms. To confirm the findings, the suspect food is again removed from the diet for several days and then reintroduced. If there is no improvement in symptoms after trying several diets, it is likely that the symptoms are not the result of food allergy or intolerance and other causes should be investigated.

Once the offending food has been identified then it can be eliminated from the diet altogether as there is no other specific treatment for food allergies.

The outlook for food allergy and food intolerance

The majority of infants and young children grow out of their allergies as they get older. For older children and adults, allergies and intolerance to certain foods tend to remain with them for the rest of their lives. For example, allergies to fish, shellfish and nuts may persist, and as reactions to them may be severe they should always be avoided.

Work being carried out in the United States offers some hope in the future for people with lifelong food allergies. This research has found that the protein molecules that trigger allergic reactions are those that are rich in disulphide bonds, that is, pairs of sulphur atoms chemically bonded together. Proteins rich in this type of disulphide bond, which are known to cause allergic reactions, include beta-lactoglobulin in milk, the 2S protein in nuts and a variety of proteins in cereals. A protein found in bacteria and some plants, thioredoxin, is known to mobilise energy reserves in these organisms by breaking down disulphide bonds. It may be possible to treat food with thioredoxin to break down the disulphide bonds and neutralise the allergens. Thioredoxin changes the shape of the offending protein so that the immune system no longer recognises or reacts against it. The protein also becomes more easily digestible so that bread and other foods derived from cereals, which are naturally rich in intact disulphide bonds, may lose their allergenic potential.

Rather than treating foods directly, it may be possible to insert the thioredoxin genes into the plants so that they grow pre-treated. This avenue of research may mean that in the future cereals and nuts may not cause allergic reactions and that milk can be treated so that everyone can drink it without adverse effects.

8

Drug Allergy

Adverse reactions to drugs are fairly common, but only a few of these reactions, probably around 5 per cent, are caused by allergy. When these reactions are allergic in nature, they may be the result of either a Type I or a Type IV reaction (*see* Chapter 1). Adverse reactions may also be caused by direct toxic effects of the drug or drug intolerance. It is estimated that up to 30 per cent of people in hospital suffer allergic reactions to drugs during treatment and that fatalities occur in about 1 in 10,000 adverse drug reactions.

Allergic symptoms in response to drugs are not only confined to atopic individuals although they, and those with debilitating diseases, do have a higher incidence of drug-induced symptoms. Women also appear to be more likely to develop drug allergies than men.

Adverse reactions to drugs may be because of toxic effects. This may be the result of an absolute overdosage because of an error in the amount or frequency of individual doses. Or it may be because of a relative overdosage as a result of the patient's body being unable to break down the drug or excrete the drug normally.

Drug intolerance may also be confused with an allergic reaction. However, there are a number of differences that distinguish one from the other. Firstly, in the case of drug intolerance, an adverse reaction develops on first use in contrast with a true allergy, when there is no adverse reaction on initial exposure. As in other allergic reactions, an adverse response develops when the drug is used on subsequent occasions. Secondly, adverse reactions in the case of drug intolerance may be either the same as would be expected to occur in a toxic reaction to a higher dose, or it may be an exaggeration of a common side effect. In allergic reactions to drugs, the symptoms and signs that develop are largely independent of the pharmacologic properties of the drug concerned.

The unexpected and peculiar adverse reactions that occur in a small proportion of people exposed to a drug are known as *idiosyncratic reactions*. Some are the result of a genetically determined enzyme deficiency, which means the person cannot break down or metabolise the drug as is normally the case. In many instances, little is known about the mechanisms by which these reactions occur.

Most toxic and idiosyncratic reactions to drugs differ sufficiently from allergic responses so as not to be confused with each other. There are a few exceptions. Some toxic and idiosyncratic reactions directly involve mast cells, causing them to release histamine. This production of allergic symptoms without the production of antibodies is sometimes known as *pseudo-allergy*. Drugs that can produce this type of reaction include some of the opiates and the contrast media or dye used in certain X-ray examinations to produce a more sharply defined image. Use of these drugs can result in the development of urticaria and, in some cases, even anaphylactic reactions.

An allergic reaction occurs only after a person has been exposed to a drug on at least one previous occasion with no adverse effect. After this initial exposure, an allergic reaction can occur in response to doses of the drug well below the usual therapeutic level. Allergic reactions to drugs usually result in a limited number of symptoms. Skin rashes (particularly urticaria), serum sickness, unexpected fever and anaphylaxis, which occur while on a course of drugs, are nearly always caused by allergy. Occasionally, cases of anaemia and thrombocytopenia are reported, and, rarely, kidney and liver damage may occur with repeated exposure.

The majority of modern synthetic drugs are made of chemicals with small molecules. In order to induce an allergic reaction, these small molecules, or their breakdown products, have to combine with larger proteins in the body. This complex of a drug molecule and protein is capable of causing antibody production and an allergic response when the drug is encountered again.

Drugs that are injected or are applied directly to the skin are more likely to provoke an allergic reaction than ones that are taken by mouth.

The list of drugs capable of causing allergic reactions

is very long. The most commonly implicated ones include penicillin and other antibiotics and aspirin preparations. Local anaesthetics, insulin, sulphonamides, codeine and barbiturates are also frequently responsible for allergies.

Penicillin and other antibiotics

Antibiotics, particularly penicillin, are the group of drugs most commonly associated with allergy. It is estimated that between 2 per cent and 5 per cent of patients treated with penicillin develop an allergic reaction. The most common symptoms are eczema, angioedema and urticaria. Ten per cent of reactions are life-threatening.

Penicillin is one member of the penicillin family of drugs. Others include ampicillin, amoxycillin, flucloxacillin, cloxacillin. These are marketed under many different names, such as Amoxil, Augmentin, Floxapen, Timentin and Magnapen. If an individual displays an allergic response to one member of the penicillin family, it is likely that he or she will respond similarly to others. It is therefore safer to avoid all members of the penicillin family, and there are many other antibiotics that can be substituted. Allergy to one antibiotic does not necessarily mean that a person will be allergic to them all. However, some patients who are allergic to penicillin may also be allergic to cephalosporins.

Studies looking at incidences of severe, even fatal, reactions to penicillin reveal that:

- about 75 per cent of patients dying of penicillin anaphylaxis had no previous history of allergic reactions to antibiotics
- in most fatal cases, the onset of allergic symptoms occurred within 60 minutes of taking the drug
- patients who experienced severe reactions other than in hospital were unconscious before medical help arrived

In common with most other drugs, the safest method of administering penicillin is by mouth. Injections are more likely to result in fatal allergic reactions.

Allergy to penicillin can wear off, and so a person who shows an allergic reaction may not be so for the rest of his or her life. Skin prick tests can be used to determine whether an allergy is still active.

Aspirin

Aspirin is a commonly used and important drug to which people may be intolerant. It was also one of the earliest drugs to be implicated in allergy and was first mentioned in this context in 1902. Aspirin was included in a publication on drug allergy in 1919.

It now appears, however, that the reaction to aspirin is not a true allergy involving the immune system. The reaction involves a response to the salicylic acid that is released from aspirin (acetyl salicylic acid). Salicylic acid stimulates mast cells directly and so causes allergic symptoms to develop. This is an example of a so-called *pseudo-allergic reaction*. IgE antibodies are not involved but the end result is the same. Aspirin is clearly associated with triggering asthma attacks. Asthmatics should avoid all forms of aspirin and aspirin-containing preparations and any drug containing salicylate, which is also likely to affect them. Many popular medicines contain aspirin, including:

Anadin	Disprin Extra
Anadin Extra	Ecotrin
Aspro	Equagesic
Asprodeine	Robaxisal
Beechams Powders	Solcode
Caprin	Solprin
Codis	Veganin
Decrin	Winsprin
Disprin	

Reaction resembling serum sickness

Serum sickness was first identified early this century and was found to be caused by horse serum used for diphtheria immunisation. Before antibiotics were discovered, infections like diphtheria and tetanus were sometimes treated by injections with horse serum. The horses from which the serum was taken had previously been injected with diphtheria and tetanus bacteria so that the serum was rich in antibodies against them. When the antibody-rich serum was injected into someone with the infection, the antibody in the serum could combat the infection and so give protection. Sometimes, particularly if serum injections were repeated, the patient developed a severe reaction, in some cases, fatal. An allergic reaction had developed to the horse serum.

Serum sickness is rarely seen these days, although serum is still used occasionally in managing diphtheria, botulism and venomous snake and spider bites. Serum from horses and other species is also used to suppress immune reactions to transplanted organs. Some drugs also cause similar symptoms. Penicillin is the drug most likely to cause this rare reaction, but sulphonamides and streptomycin have also been implicated. The allergic reaction usually appears seven to twelve days after administration of a foreign serum or drug. Reactions to foreign serum occur in at least 5 per cent of persons given it for the first time.

Serum sickness is a Type III immune reaction. The symptoms include fever, skin eruptions, including urticaria, and general aches and pains. The symptoms usually appear about seven days after receiving the substance, although they may appear sooner if the patient has been exposed previously. Sometimes there is also a mild fever but this lasts only one or two days.

Local anaesthetics

It is estimated that 5000 to 10,000 patients a year suffer an adverse reaction to commonly used anaesthetic drugs such as suxamethonium, thiopentone and alcuronium. Severe reactions occur in perhaps 300 to 500 patients per annum, with effects varying from brain damage to death.

Allergy to contact drugs

Ingredients used in topical drugs are a major cause of allergic contact dermatitis (*see* Chapter 5). Allergic contact dermatitis is a delayed hypersensitivity reaction. Drugs involved include penicillin, sulphonamides, neomycin, antihistamines, anaesthetics (benzocaine), antiseptics (thimesol, hexachlorophene) and stabilisers such as ethylerendiamine and its derivatives.

Topical sulphonamides are also implicated in photoallergic contact dermatitis, i.e. dermatitis that requires exposure to light following application of the allergic substance for the reaction to develop.

Diagnosis of drug allergy

Allergies to drugs can be diagnosed in a number of ways. When the reaction results in anaphylaxis, the drug responsible is usually easy to identify. Serum-sickness-type reactions are usually caused by penicillins, although occasionally sulphonamides, hydralazine and some other drugs may be responsible.

When a drug allergy is suspected, the taking of all medication should be suspended unless it is absolutely essential.

Skin tests can be useful in the diagnosis of the immediate type of allergic reactions such as those caused by penicillin. However, skin tests are not reliable diagnostic tools for allergies to most drugs.

Treatment of drug allergy

Most allergic reactions clear up within a few days after the drug is withdrawn. Treatment can then usually be limited to control of pain or itching.

Sometimes a drug that may be life-saving has to be continued despite allergic symptoms such as urticaria and fever. One example is the treatment of bacterial endocarditis with penicillin. In this case, urticaria can be treated with glucocorticoid as necessary.

9

Anaphylaxis and Allergy to Insects

Most allergic reactions take place locally in a particular organ or tissue, such as the nose or the lungs, and this happens when the allergen is encountered by a single organ. In some cases, however, the allergen is injected directly into the bloodstream and reaches many parts of the body at once, causing a massive reaction. This is known as an *anaphylactic reaction*. This can also occur occasionally when large doses of allergen are taken by mouth, as seen in Chapter 8.

The introduction of a toxic substance into the body usually results in the development of antibodies (usually IgG) to that toxin. When the same toxin is encountered by the body for a second time, there is some protection against it, and this is known as *prophylaxis*. When the response on a second encounter causes a more severe reaction than the first, this is known as *anaphylaxis*, that is 'no protection'. The antibodies involved here are usually IgE.

Anaphylactic reactions are the most dramatic and dangerous of all, and in some cases they can be fatal.

They usually come on very suddenly after exposure to the allergen and are often very severe, although mild reactions do sometimes occur. If the condition is recognised quickly and effective treatment given, recovery can be complete and there will be no lasting damage.

The most common causes of anaphylactic reactions are injections of drugs to which an allergy has developed and insect stings. They may also be caused by blood transfusion reactions and in response to some foods and anaesthetics. A few people can develop anaphylactic reactions following strenuous exercise; this is known as *exercise-induced anaphylaxis*.

Who is at risk?

Anaphylactic reactions are extremely rare, and even highly allergic individuals rarely experience such extreme responses. It is impossible to predict on an individual basis, but those who suffer from hay fever, asthma or other allergic conditions are generally at greater risk. The exception to this is anaphylaxis resulting from a bee or wasp sting, which can occur in individuals with no previous history of allergy. In Great Britain, about six people die each year from anaphylaxis caused by insect stings. A similar number die from anaphylactic shock after eating peanuts. All these deaths are preventable if the right medical treatment is given quickly enough. Increased public awareness of this condition may lead to fewer deaths in the future.

As with other classic allergic reactions, the first exposure to an allergen produces no ill-effect in an individual. However, this first encounter sensitises a person to
that allergen and on subsequent encounters an allergic
response can follow. A response as severe as an anaphylactic reaction happens very rarely – in the case of insect
stings, for example, fewer than 1 per cent of people who
are stung. Having once developed anaphylaxis in response to a particular allergen, a person will have a similar severe reaction every time it is encountered.

Symptoms of anaphylaxis

An anaphylactic reaction is massive, involving the
whole body. As the allergen spreads throughout the
body, it triggers off a response from mast cells in all areas. Typically, within one to fifteen minutes of receiving
the insect bite or eating the offending food, the patient
feels uneasy and becomes agitated and flushed. People
who have suffered such a reaction report that they experience a general sense of fear and dread and in some cases feel that they are going to die. This is quickly followed by a whole range of symptoms that vary from
case to case. Massive urticaria may develop, with swelling of the face, lips, tongue and throat. The pulse races,
vision may become blurred, and dizziness and faintness
develop. The patient may experience a tightness in the
throat and chest, a wheeze and may have difficulty in
breathing. Sneezing, nasal congestion and itching in the

mouth may occur, and nausea, vomiting, abdominal pain and diarrhoea are less common symptoms. Not everyone suffers all these symptoms.

In very severe cases, the manifestation of shock can develop in one to two minutes. The blood pressure falls, and the patient may suffer convulsions, become unresponsive and eventually lose consciousness. There may be a period of coma, and death sometimes follows.

If the severe acute attack is not fatal, the symptoms gradually wear off. However, the urticaria may take several weeks to disappear.

Not all anaphylactic reactions happen immediately; some take one or even two hours to develop. There are usually some signs that things are wrong, such as itching or swelling in the mouth, nausea and stomach pains.

Causes of anaphylaxis

In anaphylaxis the body mounts a dramatic response to an allergen, with the release of chemical substances from mast cells positioned throughout the body. These chemicals spread through the body via the bloodstream. Some of them act on the small blood vessels in body tissues and make them leak so that blood escapes. The leakage of blood causes swelling in the tissues. This swelling can have different effects depending upon where it occurs in the body. Swelling in the lungs causes wheezing and breathing difficulties, in the skin, redness, itching and the development of urticaria, while in the stomach, nausea and cramping pains. All parts of the body can be affected.

In some cases, because of the widespread effect of the reaction, so much fluid leaks out of the blood vessels that the total volume of blood circulating around the body decreases. This causes a drop in blood pressure and the heart has to work harder to pump enough blood around the body to serve the vital organs. The drop in blood pressure causes faintness, dizziness and, in more extreme cases, loss of consciousness.

Treatment

Immediate medical treatment is needed if death is to be avoided. The first line of treatment for anaphylaxis is an injection of adrenaline, which should be given without delay. Adrenaline counteracts the effects of the chemical mediators released by the mast cells by causing the blood vessels to contract. Sometimes antihistamines are given for milder attacks and also, in addition to adrenaline in severe attacks, to block the effects of further histamine release. Severe attacks need intensive treatment in hospital where help with breathing can be given and resuscitation equipment is available if needed.

People who have suffered one severe anaphylactic reaction are at risk of suffering another if they again encounter the same allergen. An emergency supply of adrenaline in a syringe is made available to such people to carry around with them so that they can self-administer a dose if the need arises. The emergency supply of adrenaline should be administered as soon as it is thought that a severe reaction is developing. In this situation it is better to overreact rather than wait to see what happens. There are no serious ill-effects if a dose of adrenaline is given when not strictly necessary. Adrenaline has no side effects in the doses given and is almost always completely safe. The consequences of not using it are far more devastating!

The patient should get to a hospital as soon as the adrenaline has been injected as this dose lasts for only a short time. Further doses are necessary until the condition subsides, and additional medical help may also be needed to treat the symptoms.

People who have suffered from severe anaphylactic reactions sometimes carry a medical information necklace or bracelet. This carries information about the medical condition a person suffers from and so enables appropriate medical help to be given even if the person is unconscious.

The most commonly prescribed adrenaline injection is the Epipen, which is a pre-filled syringe with a spring-loaded needle that makes it very easy to use. Instruction is given in the use of the pen, and in the case of children, other members of the family, and perhaps teachers, should also be trained in its use. The injection is usually given in the thigh, about halfway between the hip and the knee.

Some people who have experienced a serious reaction, but not severe enough to be classed as anaphylactic shock, are given adrenaline which can be administered via an inhaler similar to those used by asthmatics. One in common use is the Medihaler-Epi. By using this device, a small dose of adrenaline is inhaled into the lungs and quickly absorbed into the bloodstream. The adrenaline is then distributed throughout the body and starts working immediately. Some of the adrenaline taken in this way is absorbed directly through the mouth. As in the case of an injected dose of adrenaline, the Medihaler-Epi should be used as soon as symptoms of a severe allergic reaction begin. Antihistamines and steroid tablets may also be carried and taken when a reaction begins.

Exercise-induced anaphylaxis

This is a very unusual form of anaphylaxis. Some people who are sensitive to certain foods, say shellfish, may get relatively mild reactions when they eat this food. However, if after eating the food they then take some moderately strenuous exercise, such as running or jogging, they may suffer a severe anaphylactic reaction. In this case, the exercise acts as an additional trigger to the allergic reaction, making it much worse than the person's usual response to eating that particular food. It is not clear how or why this happens. Skin and blood tests should be made to confirm the source of the allergic reaction. The food can then be avoided in future and exercise taken without fear of anaphylaxis.

Anaphylaxis caused by drugs

A number of people are extremely allergic to some drugs and can suffer anaphylactic reactions to them. The drug that is most commonly associated with this type of reaction is penicillin. This can come in many forms and under many different trade names, as listed previously.

Allergies to insects

The most common causes of insect allergies are stings from bees and wasps. Insects that bite may inject a small amount of saliva while sucking up blood and allergies can develop to the saliva. However, allergies caused by bites and stings from insects such as ants, fleas, lice, bed bugs and mosquitoes, and also from scorpions, occur but are much less common. Occasionally inhalant and contact allergies can be caused by exposure to insect parts.

Insect stings

The honeybee and bumblebee tend to sting only when they are provoked and they die as a result. Bumblebees sting less frequently than honeybees despite their large size and noisy flight. Beekeepers are at increased risk because bees usually sting in defence of the hive. A honeybee leaves its sting in the victim, and this continues to pump out venom for some moments.

Wasps are much more aggressive insects than bees and may sting without being provoked. Wasps tend to sting repeatedly, normally using their venom to paralyse and kill insects to feed their larvae. They do not leave their sting behind in the victim.

Stinging insects deliver an injection of venom into their victim. Bee and wasp venom is a complex mixture of substances, including toxins and proteins, which can act as allergens. A sting results in a red, painful swelling around the site of injection, and sometimes this can become quite large. Multiple stings can result in the victim feeling generally unwell with fever and headache. These symptoms result from the toxin in the venom and they usually last a couple of days. Sometimes a sting can get infected and become septic. A non-allergic person can tolerate up to 500 stings from a swarm of bees.

A person who has been stung once can become sensitised to the venom and develop an allergic reaction with a subsequent sting. As the venom is injected directly into the bloodstream, an allergic reaction can develop very quickly. This response may range from relatively mild, with perhaps the development of urticaria, to very severe, resulting in an anaphylactic reaction. After a severe local response to a sting, such as a large painful lump, there is a 5 to 10 per cent chance that the next sting will provoke a severe allergic, or even anaphylactic, reaction. However, sensitisation to stings does not last a lifetime; about 50 per cent of people lose their sensitivity as time goes by.

Insect stings should be treated by removing the sting to prevent infection in the case of a bee sting and then relieving the swelling and pain by applying a cold compress to the wound. Antihistamines may be prescribed. Symptoms should subside within a few days.

The treatment for anapyhlaxis caused by insect stings has already been described. If the sting is on an arm or leg, a tourniquet can be applied as an emergency measure to try to stop the venom from spreading throughout the bloodstream and prevent the onset of an anaphylactic reaction. It should not be left in place for more than 15 minutes or until medical help is at hand. Antihistamines may be prescribed to relieve longer-term symptoms of anaphylaxis such as urticaria.

Desensitisation (allergen immunotherapy), although of dubious value in the treatment of many allergies (*see* Chapter 10), is regarded as particularly effective in the case of allergy to insect stings. A person who has experienced an anaphylactic reaction to an insect sting, has a 50 per cent chance of having a similar or worse reaction if stung again so desensitisation may be of value. The treatment involves giving regular injections, usually weekly, of venom extract. Low-concentration doses are given initially, and gradually the strength is increased. When high doses are reached, injections are given every four to six weeks for at least two years and for perhaps as long as five years. Desensitisation gives a 90 per cent protection against further anaphylactic reactions to insect stings.

In 1986, stringent restrictions were put on this form of treatment because of the increasing number of severe adverse reactions to desensitisation, including several deaths. Such treatments can now be carried out only in specialist allergy clinics following very strict guidelines. The treatment is allowed only for certain groups of people and usually not for children.

For someone who is at risk of a severe reaction to a sting, the best course of action for him or her is to take measures to avoid contact with the insects. Such measures include:

- avoiding beehives and wasps' nests or areas where these may be present
- always wearing shoes outdoors when insects may be around
- keeping rubbish areas clean and tidy
- taking care when eating or drinking while out of doors in the summer
- wearing insect repellent while out of doors in the summer
- not wearing perfumes, aftershaves or cosmetics with strong fragrances that attract insects.
- keeping car and house windows shut, especially in the late summer when wasps can be a greater problem

Above all, people should not panic when there are bees and wasps around; flapping arms can provoke them into stinging.

Inhalant allergies caused by insects

Minute parts of insects, such as shed skin scales, faecal particles and dried body secretions, are often found as constituents of house dust. When inhaled by sensitised people, these can cause symptoms of inhalant allergies such as rhinitis and asthma. The house dust mite is an important cause of allergic symptoms of asthma, as has been described in Chapter 3. Other insects, such as aphids, weevils, cockroaches, locusts and green nimitti flies, can all cause similar allergic conditions.

The green nimitti fly (*Chironomus lewisi*), a type of midge, has been a major cause of symptoms of asthma and hay fever in areas of northern Africa such as the Sudan and Egypt. These non-biting flies are often found swarming by water at dusk. The allergy is caused by the inhalation of minute fragments of the insect's body, and people allergic to one species often react to others as well. The larvae of one species, *Chironomus riparius*, is used as food for pet fish, and there have been cases of rhinitis in Europe as a result of exposure to fish food.

Contact allergies

Contact with various species of hairy caterpillar can cause a condition called *caterpillar urticaria*. This may cause severe eruptions of the skin and mouth. The condition can be treated with antihistamines, cold compresses and painkillers.

10

Diagnosis and Tests for Allergies

Accurate diagnosis of an allergy is important so that improvements in health and, in some cases, a cure can be achieved. The cause of many allergies is obvious. When the symptoms appear either immediately or very shortly after exposure to an allergen it can be easy to pinpoint what is causing the symptoms. For example, if the eyes start streaming and the nose begins to run shortly after walking through a field on a fine summer's day, it can be fairly certain that these symptoms are caused by pollen in the air. This can be confirmed if the symptoms disappear soon after going indoors, away from the pollen. Similarly, if a person comes out in a rash every time he or she eats shellfish, the cause of the allergy is obvious. No further investigations are necessary – the symptoms can be cured by avoiding the allergen. However, there are a number of allergic conditions in which the cause is not so obvious. This is the case especially where exposure to the allergen is continuous or frequent, for example, allergy to certain basic foods or an airborne substance in the environment. In these cases, there may be a need, firstly, to determine whether the symptoms are allergic in nature and, secondly, the source of the allergen.

Diagnosis of an allergic condition, as with any medical condition, can be made by a combination of assessing the symptoms, examining the patient and carrying out certain diagnostic tests.

Case histories and diaries

Both case histories and diaries of symptoms can reveal a great deal of information about an individual's allergies. They can reveal when the allergy first appeared, whether the symptoms are seasonal, whether they occur after being in particular environments and whether they disappear when there is a change of surroundings, e.g. on a visit abroad, when not at work, etc. Information on whether the symptoms appear or get worse when a person is under stress, takes exercise or after some other trigger can also be helpful. All this sort of information helps to build up a picture of the allergy and its symptoms and to pinpoint the source.

Skin tests

Skin tests have been used for a long time as the principal method of detecting substances responsible for producing allergic symptoms. The skin contains mast cells, which, like those in the nose or lungs, are primed to react to allergens. When an allergen is introduced into the skin, the mast cells are induced to produce histamine and other chemicals and so produce an allergic reaction. Skin tests are most reliable in confirming allergies to inhaled substances, but they can also be useful where food, insects or anaesthetics are suspected of being the culprits. There are three types of test that are used: the skin prick test, intradermal testing and patch testing.

Skin prick test

This is probably the most commonly used allergy test. It is most reliable in identifying airborne allergies but less so in food allergies, particularly where milk, cereal or grains are involved. (Exclusion diets are a better method for diagnosing food allergies, *see* Chapter 7).

The test consists of making a tiny prick with a needle or lance through a droplet of the allergen placed on the skin. This is done very gently so as not to draw blood. The test is usually carried out on the back or on the skin of the inner forearm. When the patient being tested is an infant, the skin on the back is most commonly used. A number of allergens can be tested at one time, and the skin is marked to identify the site of each test. Clean needles are used to test each allergen to avoid cross-contamination.

A small amount of the extract seeps through to the lower layers of the skin, and if the person is allergic a typical weal and flare reaction is observed. This consists of a reddening and swelling (the weal) around the area of the skin prick. There may also be some itching. This reaction usually develops within ten minutes. A weal greater than 2 mm in diameter, sometimes 3 mm, is considered a positive reaction to the allergen. The symptoms of this reaction subside within a couple of hours.

Positive and negative controls are carried out at the same time. A negative control consists of a drop of saline solution on the skin, which is pricked in the same way as the other allergens to be tested. No one should react to this test, although some very sensitive people react to any minor skin trauma. If there is a reaction to the control, then doubt is cast on the results of the skin prick tests. It can be concluded that any other positive reactions may also be caused by the irritant effect alone. A positive control solution contains histamine, to which everyone should react. A negative reaction to this test may be because the patient is receiving certain medication, e.g. antihistamines, corticosteroids or certain antidepressant drugs. The person carrying out the test should be informed if the patient is on any such drugs as this may render the test results unreliable.

A negative skin prick test means that the patient is almost certainly not allergic to that particular substance. However, not everyone who has a positive reaction may display symptoms of allergy. A positive result may indicate that the person has a latent allergy, i.e. he or she is sensitised to an allergen but is not exhibiting allergic symptoms. A positive test indicates that a patient has the *potential* to develop an allergy and may develop symptoms later in life.

The skin prick test is a very sensitive diagnostic tool. This can be illustrated by the test for platinum allergy in which it has been calculated that as few as 200,000 molecules of a platinum salt will give a positive reaction. It is also a relatively cheap and easy test to administer and that is why it is the first to be employed in diagnosing allergy. The skin prick test is extremely safe and should be risk-free – even the most sensitive person does not normally experience a bad reaction. It is almost painless and well tolerated even by infants. However, in some elderly people the skin may not be capable of reacting and so skin testing in this group is of no value.

It is important that the test is administered by a properly qualified person, firstly to make sure that the test is carried out and interpreted correctly, and secondly to ensure that, on the extremely rare occasions that a severe reaction occurs, appropriate help is available.

Intradermal testing

Intradermal tests are sometimes used when skin prick tests show a negative result but strong suspicions remain that a particular substance is causing an allergy. The test consists of injecting a small amount of a dilute allergen extract into the skin, using a fine needle and syringe. A positive reaction is similar to that caused by the skin prick test and consists of swelling, itching and a raised blister-like weal. The reaction usually develops within about 10 to 20 minutes and disappears again in one to two hours.

Sometimes this type of test can provoke a severe response and there is a risk of an anaphylactic reaction. For this reason, the test is rarely used in Britain although it is still widely used in the United States. It is also not considered very reliable, as it can give false positive results caused by injecting a relatively high concentration of allergen which can indicate an allergy where none in fact exists.

Patch testing

A patch test is a special type of skin test used in the diagnosis of eczema or dermatitis as a result of allergy. This type of allergy is caused by T lymphocytes and not IgE antibodies. The reactions are therefore delayed, and so allergic contact eczema is a chronic condition rather than occurring in acute attacks. This test is also useful for allergens that cannot readily be dissolved in a liquid.

Patch tests use a series of discs, about the size of a one pence piece, which are impregnated with a small amount of the suspected allergen in soft paraffin (Vaseline). The discs are then applied to the skin, usually on the back, and are kept in place by a hypo-allergenic adhesive dressing for 48 hours, during which time they must be kept dry. While the disc is in place the allergen seeps through the skin. When the discs are removed, any redness or swelling is noted and the test area is re-examined in another 48 hours.

Although patch testing is simple in principle, it needs to be carried out by an expert, as getting the correct dose of allergen is vital to achieve a good result. Accurate interpretation of positive results also requires a great deal of skill and experience. Some of the substances being tested may themselves cause irritant effects that can be confused with an allergic response.

Patch tests are relatively simple, safe and inexpensive, and are particularly useful for all forms of contact dermatitis. Although allergic reactions to substances can be detected in this way, discovering how the patient is exposed to the allergen may take further investigations. For example, positive patch tests to chrome, in patients suffering from dermatitis caused by cement, were considered puzzling but irrelevant until it was eventually shown that cement contains minute amounts of chrome salts.

Blood tests

Blood tests are increasingly used for allergy diagnosis. A small quantity of blood can be used to identify the antibodies involved in allergic reactions. People with allergies often have increased levels of IgE antibodies in their blood, but this may also be caused by other factors.

RAST (radio-allergosorbent test)
This test is used to measure the amount of IgE antibody against individual allergens, e.g. grass pollen or house

dust mite. A small sample of blood is taken, usually from a vein in the arm. The sample is then sent to a specialist laboratory where the test is carried out. A radioactive label is introduced, which attaches itself to the IgE antibody against a particular allergen present in the blood sample. This is done by attaching very pure extracts of the allergen to the surface of a paper disc. The blood sample is added to the disc and if it contains IgE antibodies to that particular allergen, they will attach themselves to it. The next step is to add a special antibody against IgE, which is labelled with a radioisotope. If any IgE has stuck to the allergen then the radioactive anti-IgE will bind itself on as well. Levels of the radioactive-labelled anti-IgE can be measured using a radioactive counter. This is very sensitive, and even very low levels of IgE can be measured. The amount of IgE antibody in the patient's blood can be estimated from this measure of radioactivity. (*See* Fig. 10.1)

RAST does not have any advantages over skin tests, which are probably more sensitive. However, it is often used in conjunction with a skin test if the result of the latter is not conclusive. RAST can also be used when skin tests cannot be carried out, for example, on children who have severe eczema. It is also particularly useful if there is a risk of an anaphylactic reaction to a skin test, or if a patient is on antihistamines that cannot be withdrawn.

Skin tests are fast, cheap and reliable. RAST is safe but more expensive, and the involvement of specialist

Figure 10.1: The Rast test

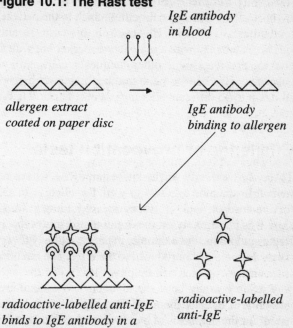

*IgE antibody
in blood*

*allergen extract
coated on paper disc*

*IgE antibody
binding to allergen*

*radioactive-labelled anti-IgE
binds to IgE antibody in a
positive test*

*radioactive-labelled
anti-IgE*

laboratories to carry out the tests means that it may take several days for the results to be known. RAST is not helpful to test for food allergy. A negative RAST result does not completely rule out the possibility that the patient is allergic to that particular allergen. False negative results do sometimes occur.

MAST (multiple allergosorbent test)

In this test, the anti-IgE antibodies attach to the patient's antibodies as in RAST. However, in this case the anti-IgE is not labelled with a radioactive marker but with an enzyme that reacts with other chemicals, causing luminescence. This can be photographed using high-speed film. Up to 35 different allergens can be detected in one test.

Challenge or provocation tests

These are used only when skin tests or RAST have not helped in diagnosing the cause of the allergy. In this test, instead of applying the suspected allergen to the skin, it is put directly on the organ that displays the allergic symptoms. For example, in the case of hay fever a particular pollen is introduced to the nose. The intention is that the symptoms will be provoked in just the same way as they would be if the allergen was encountered naturally in the environment. This type of test is most useful for the diagnosis of hay fever and asthma but it is also used in food allergy.

Nasal challenge

This is particularly useful in determining the cause of allergy in the case of perennial rhinitis. The cause of seasonal rhinitis (hay fever) is often obvious (*see* Chapter 3), but the cause of perennial rhinitis is often not so clear cut. It may be useful in determining which constituent of house dust the patient is allergic to, e.g. the house dust mite, animal dander or cat fur.

In this test a small quantity of suspect allergen extract is sprayed up the nose. This is performed just after the patient has breathed in to prevent the allergen, e.g. a pollen, getting into the lungs and perhaps provoking an asthma attack. If the person is allergic, the response is usually immediate. The results of the test can be assessed by observing the symptoms of hay fever that occur, including sneezing, nasal blockage, a watery discharge and itching. The inside of the nose can also be examined to observe the changes in inflammation. In addition, the nasal resistance to airflow before and after the test can be measured using a simple nasal inspiratory flow meter (SNIF meter).

The results of this test can be affected if the patient is on certain medications such as antihistamines or steroid sprays. The patient should stop taking these for a period before having the provocation test.

Bronchial challenge

This test involves inhaling the suspected allergen and is often carried out using a nebuliser (*see* Chapter 3). The response is measured using the lung function tests described in Chapter 3. The concentrations of the suspected allergen can be increased until there is a predetermined drop in lung function. At this point the chest may feel a little tight and wheezy but the symptoms should be mild. Lung function is returned to normal by using a bronchodilator.

This type of test is used very rarely, but it can be useful in the diagnosis of asthma caused by workplace exposure to allergens. It can also be useful when a measurable response to an allergen is required, for example, to find out whether one drug is more suitable than another or to determine if someone's asthma improves when he or she stops working with a particular substance.

As there is a risk of a severe anaphylactic reaction in a small number of patients, this test is only carried out in hospital. There is sometimes a delayed reaction to the allergen so the patient must be kept under observation for up to 48 hours.

Oral challenge tests (food challenges)

Distinguishing allergies caused by food is difficult as the symptoms are often not clear cut and skin tests are usually unhelpful. If a particular dietary substance is suspected of causing an allergy, a food challenge test may help. The first step in this type of test requires that the food under suspicion must be totally eliminated from the diet for a period of time. If the symptoms disappear, the food is reintroduced to see if this prompts them to recur. The food being reintroduced is contained in a gelatine capsule so that it cannot be tasted and the patient does not know the contents. Any reaction is then noted. After an interval of three days, the process is repeated but with a totally non-allergic food in an identical capsule – this is the placebo, or dummy. Neither the patient nor the doctor knows which capsule contains the suspect food or which is the dummy. This is known as a double blind test, and it aims to eliminate bias and subjectivity on the part of the doctor or patient. The whole process can be repeated with several different foods.

A double blind food challenge is extremely reliable and if an allergy is present, symptoms will appear when the food responsible is introduced. However, if no symptoms occur allergy cannot be ruled out. This may be because giving the suspect allergen in such a test is not the same as a continuous exposure to the food over a long period, which is probably how it is taken in normal circumstances.

It is essential that this type of food challenge test is performed by an expert with medical help at hand because of the risk of an anaphylactic reaction. It should never be given to someone who has already experienced such a reaction.

Lung function tests

There are two forms of lung function test commonly used to diagnose asthma: one is called the peak expiratory volume (PEV) and the other the peak expiratory flow rate (PEFR). They both involve blowing air as hard as possible through the mouthpiece of measuring equipment. Peak expiratory flow volume involves measuring how quickly and efficiently the lungs can be emptied. This requires the use of a spirometer, a relatively expensive and bulky piece of equipment, and so this test is rarely done outside a hospital. Measurement of the peak expiratory flow rate can be performed using an inexpensive piece of equipment, a peak flow meter, and can be carried out at home. More details of this test can be found in Chapter 3.

The peak flow meter can give a reliable and objective measure of how easily air can pass in and out of the lungs. It is therefore useful not only in diagnosing asthma but also in monitoring changes in the condition, especially in relation to the use of medication. (*See* Chapter 3).

Bowel biopsy

This test is used as confirmation of a suspected food allergy in infant colitis and also in the diagnosis of coeliac disease. A small piece of the lining of the bowel is removed and examined under the microscope. In the case of allergic infant colitis, the biopsy can confirm the inflammation of the bowel lining and, in the case of coeliac disease, the amount of damage.

The biopsy can be carried out using one of two methods. The first method involves passing a fibre-optic tube via the mouth to the stomach and small intestine. A small sample of the bowel lining is removed. This method is usually used in adults. The second method is similar, but in this case a small capsule called a Crosby capsule is passed into the small intestine attached to a fine hollow tube. Use of an X-ray confirms when the capsule is in the correct position, and it is then fired to take a sample of the lining and the tube is then removed. This method is usually used in children. A sedative is often given to help patients relax while the tube is passed into the stomach and small intestine.

Confirmation of a diagnosis of coeliac disease is important as the only treatment for this condition is the complete avoidance of gluten and all foods containing it (*see* Chapter 7). A change to a strict gluten-free diet is something that should be undertaken only if absolutely necessary.

11

Autoimmune Diseases

One of the prime characteristics of the immune system is its ability to recognise 'self' so that it does not react against its own body tissues. In some individuals this ability is defective or breaks down and autoimmune diseases are the result. In this group of diseases the immune system fails to recognise its own body tissues and produces antibodies to antigens within the body, resulting in damage.

In the Gell and Coombs classification of hypersensitivity reactions, as described in Chapter 1, autoimmune diseases are classified as Type III reactions, i.e. those resulting from the deposition of soluble circulating antigen-antibody immune complexes in blood vessels or tissues.

Many diseases are caused by self-destructive processes, and none of the body's organs or systems is safe from possible attack. Autoimmune disease is not well understood, but it is believed that in most people the immune system is capable of producing antibodies against itself. In the majority of people this process is kept under control and no adverse symptoms are expressed.

Autoimmune diseases develop in those individuals in whom the control mechanism is not functioning properly.

It was not until the 1950s that autoimmune diseases became widely recognised. Since then the list of diseases that are thought to be the result of autoimmune causes has grown rapidly. Table 11.1 lists some of these diseases.

There are also a number of other inflammatory diseases for which there is no other reasonable explanation for their cause.

Some autoimmune diseases affect one organ or system while others affect several and are sometimes referred to as *non-organ specific*. The diseases in the latter category include systemic lupus erythematosus (SLE), rheumatoid arthritis, Sjögren's syndrome and scleroderma.

What causes autoimmune diseases?

Autoimmunity can be caused by abnormalities or defects in almost any part of the immune process. Development of these diseases in individuals is thought to be the result of the interplay of a number of complex factors involving the immune system, genetic predisposition and environmental factors.

Table 11.1: Diseases suspected of being auto-immune in origin

Highly probable	Goodpasture's syndrome Systemic lupus erythematosus Hashimoto's thyroiditis (underactive thyroid) Graves' disease (overactive thyroid) Autoimmune haemolytic anaemia Pemphigus Myasthenia gravis Multiple sclerosis Autoimmune thrombocytopaenia (low platelet levels)
Probable	Diabetes mellitus (some) Myositis Rheumatoid arthritis Sjögren's syndrome Scleroderma Pernicious anaemia
Possible	Primary biliary cirrhosis Chronic active hepatitis Vasculitis Vitiglio Urticaria, atopic dermatitis, some cases of asthma

Immune system involvement in autoimmune diseases

In patients with autoimmune diseases, such as rheumatoid arthritis and Sjögren's disease, increased numbers of a particular type of B cell (CD5) are found. These B cells have been found to produce antibodies that bind to DNA and produce rheumatoid factors.

Overproduction and underproduction of another cell of the immune system, the T cells, are also implicated in autoimmune disease. T suppressor cells are important in the recognition of 'self' and 'non-self' and therefore play an important role in preventing autoimmune disease. There is some evidence that patients with these diseases have poorly functioning T suppressor cells and their immune systems are not able to regulate the response to antigens, whether they be 'foreign' or 'self'. Lower numbers of T suppressor cells along with decreased cell activity have been reported in patients with autoimmune conditions. However, some healthy individuals also have poorly functioning T suppressor cells, and so there is more than this factor involved.

An elevated level of another T cell, the T helper cell, is thought to be involved in an excess production of self-antigens, leading to increased susceptibility to autoimmune disease.

Inherited defects in components of the complement system, which are involved in dissolving antigen-antibody complexes, may also contribute to the development of autoimmune diseases.

Other factors involved in autoimmune disease

It is not clear why some individuals suffer from autoimmune diseases while others, who are often very closely related, do not. It appears that a number of factors are important in determining whether autoimmune disease will develop. Perhaps the most important of these is a genetic predisposition to develop such a disease. In individuals with an inherited tendency, a number of environmental factors may then provoke the development of the disease. These environmental factors include infection with bacteria or viruses, diet, stress and tissue injury, such as occurs with exposure to ultraviolet light. Women are much more likely to develop autoimmune disorders than men, and it is therefore likely that hormonal influences are also important. Abnormalities in enzymes in the blood are also implicated, particularly in the haemolytic anaemias.

It is likely that a combination of these factors needs to be present for a particular autoimmune disease to develop. Also, it may be the specific combinations of these factors that lead to such a wide range of diseases.

Some of the more common autoimmune diseases are described more fully in the next section.

Systemic lupus erythematosus (SLE)

This disease is a classic autoimmune disease mainly affecting women (over 90 per cent of cases) in their child-bearing years although it can also affect children. Patients who suffer from this disease have abnormalities throughout their immune system.

The course of the disease can vary widely, depending on the degree of inflammation and organs involved. Symptoms can last for years, although there can be periods, stretching into years, of remission. Women do not usually suffer flare-ups of the condition after the menopause. With early and accurate diagnosis, so that the early stages of the disease can be controlled, prospects for long-term survival are good.

Symptoms

Symptoms include skin rashes, particularly where the skin is exposed to the light. These range from minor red discolorations to large blisters. There is also joint pain and swelling of the joints, and in some cases these may become deformed because of inflammation. The patient also suffers from severe fatigue, which can be very disabling. The inflammation associated with SLE may also affect the heart and lungs and can make breathing difficult where there is a build-up of fluid. The central nervous system may also be affected, resulting in a variety of symptoms ranging from migraines to epileptic fits. Kidney damage is found in a number of patients with SLE. The more severe the kidney involvement, the less likely the patients are to survive in the long term.

SLE may also be responsible for the destruction of red and white blood cells and platelets. This drastically reduces the body's immune defences, leaving patients prone to infection, anaemia and bruising.

Autoimmune features

Patients usually have a range of different antibodies circulating in their blood, including an autoantibody to DNA. Immune complexes of DNA and anti-DNA antibodies are formed in the circulation and are deposited in body tissues. This starts a chain of inflammatory events that results in kidney damage. Measurement of DNA antibody levels and complement in the blood are used to monitor the progress of the disease.

Treatment

There is no cure for SLE, but the symptoms can usually be controlled successfully. Milder cases may require little or no therapy. Nonsteroid anti-inflammatory agents can be used and anti-malarial drugs are useful in reducing joint pain, lethargy and skin rashes.

In more severe cases, especially when the heart and lungs are involved, steroids are used to control symptoms. Use of steroids does carry side effects, including: thinning of the bones, diabetes mellitus, high blood pressure and an increased risk of infection. In some cases a combination of drugs, including steroids, azathioprine and cyclophosphamide, may be used.

Plasmapheresis, or plasma exchange, is another treatment that may be used for patients with SLE. In this treatment, blood from the patient, is removed via a vein and passed through a machine that separates the components of the blood. The part of the blood containing the antibodies, the plasma, is removed in an attempt to halt the autoimmune process and to let the immunosuppressive drugs get the upper hand. This is a very expensive procedure and not always successful in the longer term as some patients experience a resurgence of symptoms after a few weeks.

Rheumatoid arthritis

This is an inflammatory condition that can affect a number of body systems but it principally attacks the small joints of the hands and feet. Other joints can also be involved, including the elbows, shoulders, knees and hips. It is the synovial membrane in these joints, which is responsible for lubricating them, that is affected by the inflammation. The joints become dry and damaged, causing swelling and pain. Women are two to three times more commonly affected than men. Onset of the condition may be at any age but is usually between the ages of 30 and 55. The condition can last for several years.

Symptoms
Onset of the condition may be abrupt, with inflammation of many joints simultaneously, but progressive involvement of joints is more common. The condition can range from relatively mild to very severe, with the joints

becoming deformed, and there is little effective treatment available. The majority of patients suffer a chronic, persistent condition that results in a slow destruction of the joints and erosion of the underlying bone.

All the involved joints become very tender, and this is the most sensitive physical sign of the disease. Thickening of the joints is the most specific physical sign and usually in a symmetric fashion. Joint stiffness when getting up in the morning or after prolonged inactivity is common. Fatigue and a general feeling of malaise may also occur.

Other symptoms may accompany rheumatoid arthritis, including weight loss, thinning of the skin with increased risk of ulceration, dryness of the eyes and/or mouth and, in some cases, inflammation of the peripheral nerves causing numbness in the hands and feet. One very serious complication of this condition that occurs occasionally is the rare case when the first and second joints of the spine are affected. The thickening that forms between these joints presses on the spinal cord and can cause paralysis of the arms and legs. Modern surgery can usually help before these serious consequences are realised.

Autoimmune features

Patients with rheumatoid arthritis have an antibody, IgM, circulating in their blood, known as the rheumatoid factor, which binds with another antibody, IgG. High levels of IgM are found in patients with rheumatoid arthritis but increased quantities are also found in a number of other infections and malignancies. It is believed that these antibody complexes are implicated in the immunological damage to the joints.

Treatment

The condition in up to 70 per cent of patients improves with conservative treatment in their first year of disease, but 10 per cent are eventually disabled in spite of extensive intervention.

Bed rest, particularly in the most active and painful stages of severe disease, is often helpful. A few patients also find that changes in their diet may help their condition, as may dietary supplements with fish and plant oils.

The traditional treatment for rheumatoid arthritis has been with aspirin-type drugs (salicylates), which are a relatively safe, inexpensive, anti-inflammatory form of therapy and do offer some relief. A number of people show adverse reactions to aspirin, including irritation of the gastrointestinal tract, and so it is not suitable for everyone.

A range of nonsteroidal anti-inflammatory drugs (NSAIDs) can also be used. These include Ibuprofen, Indoemthacin, Fenoprofen and Flurbiprofen. Adverse side effects of these include gastric symptoms and gastrointestinal bleeding.

Gold compounds may also be given in addition to salicylates or NSAIDs if the latter do not give adequate relief on their own. Penicillamine is also used, but side effects are more common and may give rise to kidney damage and bone marrow suppression.

Steroids have the most dramatic short-term effects on the disease, but their effect diminishes after prolonged use and they also have serious side effects.

Cytotoxic or immunosuppressive drugs such as methotrexate and azathioprine are increasingly used in severe cases of rheumatoid arthritis. These drugs are sometimes known as disease-modifying, but their mode of operation is not clear. They can suppress inflammation and relieve pain and so reduce the levels of steroid drugs that have to be used. There are major side effects with all of them, including liver disease, bone marrow suppression and possible increased risk of malignancy, particularly in relation to long-term use of axathioprine.

Sjögren's syndrome

This disorder is characterised by dryness of the mouth, eyes and other mucous membranes. It is often associated with other autoimmune conditions such as rheumatoid arthritis and SLE. About a third of patients with Sjögren's syndrome also have rheumatoid symptoms, but these tend to be mild and do not lead to destruction of the joints. In severe cases the dryness of the eye can lead to damage of the cornea. As with most autoimmune diseases, this condition is more common in women than men.

In patients with this condition, the salivary glands in the mouth, the lachrymal glands in the eyes and various others throughout the body, which are responsible for keeping membranes moist, are infiltrated with cells of the immune system. These cells, mostly macrophages and lymphocytes, lead to the destruction of the glands' ability to secrete mucous. High levels of immune complexes are also found circulating in patients' blood.

The disease is usually treated symptomatically with the use of eye-drops, mouthwashes and lubricants for other mucous tissues affected. Occasionally treatment with steroids is prescribed.

Scleroderma

This condition usually begins with the skin of the fingers and hands becoming hardened and thickened and the circulation becomes restricted (known as Raynaud's syndrome). The disease can spread rapidly to involve the arms, the chest and, in some cases, the legs as well. The skin becomes shiny and taut and may lose colour. The joints may become affected, and in severe cases, the skin around the mouth may become so dry and hard that it is difficult to eat.

In more severe cases the internal organs may also be affected, particularly the oesophagus, the intestinal tract, the lungs, the heart and the kidneys. In the case of the kidneys, the disease may be life-threatening.

Several types of autoantibodies have been identified

in patients with this condition but their role in the development of the disease is not clear.

The course of the disease is variable and unpredictable, and there have been some cases of spontaneous remission. Often the disease remains limited and does not progress to involve serious symptoms. Women are four times more likely to suffer from scleroderma than men and it is comparatively rare in children.

There is no effective treatment for the disease but the symptoms can be controlled and relieved using a variety of drugs.

Autoimmune thyroid disease

There are two forms of autoimmune thyroid disease, one associated with overproduction of the thyroid hormone, Graves' disease, and the other with a reduction in the level of hormone produced, Hashimoto's disease (also known as myxoedema).

The thyroid gland is situated at the back of the neck, and the hormone it produces, thyroxine, is important in a range of metabolic processes in the body. It is essential for the normal functioning of muscles, bone growth and mental function. It is believed that antibodies or antibody complexes infiltrate cells in the thyroid and these are later killed by killer lymphocyte cells.

Hashimoto's disease underproduction of thyroxine leads to lethargy, dry skin and hair, and damage to the nerves in the limbs. Patients require lifelong replacement of the thyroid hormone. Hashimoto's disease is eight times more prevalent in women than men, and onset occurs most often between the ages of 30 and 50. There is often a family history of thyroid disorders.

Graves' disease, caused by overproduction of thyroxine, leads to weight loss, anxiety, tremor of the hands and often a fast pulse rate. Patients with this condition also have protruding eyeballs, a very distinctive feature. They are also usually very sensitive to heat and suffer from increased sweating. This condition is seven more times likely to occur in women than men, and onset usually occurs in patients in their forties.

Patients with Graves' disease have antibodies that bind to, and stimulate, hormone receptors on the thyroid gland. Thus the autoantibodies lead the thyroid to overproduce thyroxine.

Insulin-dependent diabetes mellitus (IDDM)

There are two types of diabetes but only Type I is autoimmune in origin. In this type, autoantibodies target the insulin-producing cells of the pancreas, the beta-cells, and over a period of five to ten years all these cells are killed. Symptoms do not manifest themselves until about 90 per cent of the cells are destroyed.

Without insulin, excess levels of sugar build up, particularly in the blood, and the body works overtime to try and deal with this. This results in the clinical manifestations of the disease, including excessive thirst and the passing of increasing amounts of dilute, sugary urine. There is also a loss of weight and a feeling of weakness, and vision may become blurred and misty. If the condition persists without treatment, it can lead to diabetic coma and death. Damage to the kidneys, blood vessels and central nervous system can also occur and may be difficult to treat.

The traditional treatment for IDDM is injections two or three times a day with insulin. This insulin is mainly derived from animal sources, although more recently genetically engineered human sources have been tried with varying success.

IDDM usually develops in young people between the ages of 10 and 20 years, although it can occur at any age. There is a strong genetic predisposition to the disease, as indicated by the fact that if one identical twin develops IDDM then there is a 40–50 per cent chance that the other will also be affected.

Pernicious anaemia

This is a relatively common condition that mainly affects middle-aged women. The main symptom of this disease is weakness but sometimes numbness in the hands and feet also occurs.

Patients with this condition have antibodies to some of the cells lining the stomach, including the binding sites for vitamin B_{12}, so absorption of this important substance is impaired and a characteristic anaemia with enlarged red blood cells develops. This disease can be successfully treated with regular injections of vitamin B_{12}.

Autoimmune haemolytic anaemia and thrombocytopenia

Haemolytic anaemia is the breakdown of red blood cells because of the formation of antibodies against them. This condition may occur on its own but is often found in patients suffering with systemic lupus erythematosus. Patients with this form of anaemia feel extremely tired and exhausted and have a pale complexion. If the condition becomes severe it can lead to death.

Thrombocytopenia is also the result of an autoimmune attack on another type of red blood cell – the platelets – which are important in blood clotting. Patients with this condition have very low levels of platelets, which results in the skin and internal organs bruising and bleeding more easily.

Both these conditions can be treated with steroids, often in high doses. Other immunosuppressive drugs may also be prescribed.

Goodpasture's syndrome

This is an uncommon Type II hypersensitivity condition of unknown cause. It occurs most often in young men.

In this condition antibodies to the cells that line the kidney (and sometimes the lung) are formed. Immune complexes are formed in these organs and the complement system is activated (see Chapter 1). At the same time, lymphocytes and macrophages are attracted to these tissues, which causes inflammation and damage. Kidney damage may result, and this may lead rapidly to death if treatment is not administered promptly.

Treatment for this disease relies on the use of high doses of steroids together with immunosuppressive drugs and repeated plasma exchange to remove the offending circulating antibody.

Multiple sclerosis

This is a slowly progressive disease of the central nervous system that is characterised by the removal of layers of the white myelin sheath that surrounds the nerves. This process is known as *demyelination* and occurs in patches along the nerves. Myelin is responsible for the rapid transmission of nervous impulses around the body. Demyelination reduces the effectiveness of nerve transmission and is the cause of the symptoms associated with multiple sclerosis, including muscle weakness, progressive paralysis and the loss of feeling in different parts of the skin. Patients with this condition often experience periods of remission, often lasting months or years. However, these periods of remission grow progressively shorter until permanent disablement occurs.

The condition is usually not life-threatening and the average illness lasts more than 25 years, although the course of the disease is highly variable and unpredictable.

The cause of multiple sclerosis is unknown, but it is believed to be an autoimmune condition. T cells and macrophages are found in the patches of demyelination along the nerves. However, several other possible explanations have also been put forward – for example that it is caused by a latent virus although none has been identified.

Women are more often affected by multiple sclerosis than men, and the disease is more common in temperate climates than in the tropics. Although the age of onset is usually between the ages of 20 and 40 years, the occurrence of the disease is linked to the geographic area in which the patient spends the first 15 years of life. Moving to a different area after this age does not alter the risk of contracting this disease.

There is no specific treatment, but steroids can reduce the duration of an acute attack and hasten recovery and so help avoid permanent neurological damage. Patients should avoid overwork and fatigue.

12

Immunodeficiency Diseases

This is another group of diseases caused by the malfunctioning of the immune system. In this case, a defect in the immune system means that it is not able to protect the body against invading foreign agents, as would normally be the case. One or more parts of the immune system may be involved.

This diverse group of conditions is characterised by an increased susceptibility to infection, and individuals with such diseases may suffer severe, acute, recurrent or chronic disease. Immunodeficiency should be considered in all patients who suffer from recurrent episodes of infection. The recognition of such a deficiency of the immune system may be overlooked because of the widespread use of antibiotics in treating infection.

Immunodeficiency diseases can be categorised into two distinct groups distinguished by the nature of the origin of the disease. The first group, the *primary immune deficiency diseases* (also known as *innate immune deficiency*), is genetic in origin. The condition is present from birth, although it is often not recognised at that time as there may be no obvious manifestations. Children are partly protected from infection in their first year of life by antibodies that pass from the mother to the foetus and by those present in breast milk. The immunodeficiency usually becomes apparent over the first few years of life. There are now over 70 conditions classified as primary immunodeficient diseases. The frequency of these diseases is estimated at 1 in every 10,000 of the population – about 70 per cent of cases occur in males. Although these are rare conditions and are of limited significance on a global scale, they have been important in increasing knowledge and understanding of the development of the immune system and in demonstrating the roles played by specific genes and immune pathways.

In the past five years, the genetic cause of many of these diseases has been confirmed with the discovery of the gene that has been responsible for the condition. This has led to changes in the way in which the diseases are managed and treated, including genetic counselling for the families involved.

The second category of immunodeficiency diseases is known as *secondary* or *acquired immune deficiency diseases*. These are caused by the impairment of the immune system resulting from illnesses in previously normal individuals. They may also arise after a course of drugs, particularly immunosuppressive agents, or after exposure to chemicals toxic to the immune system. The impairment may be reversible if the underlying condition or illness can be rectified.

The secondary immune deficiency diseases are more common than the primary ones. Common causes of the second group of diseases include malnutrition, stress, burns, certain autoimmune disorders, such as diabetes mellitus and lupus erythematosus (*see* Chapter 11), and some viruses. Patients using steroid drugs over long periods are also at increased risk of immunodeficiency diseases. However, transplant and cancer patients probably comprise the largest group of patients. Transplant patients take immunosuppressant drugs to reduce the risk of the graft being rejected. Likewise, many of the drugs used to treat cancer patients are also potent immunosuppressants. Use of these drugs often impairs the normal working of the immune system. However, the most prominent group of patients with immunodeficiency diseases are those patients with Aids (Acquired Immune Deficiency Syndrome), which occurs as a secondary infection in patients infected with HIV (the Human Immunodeficiency Virus).

Primary immunodeficiency

Primary immunodeficiency diseases may be caused by defects in the B cells, the T cells, the phagocytic cells or in the complement system (*see* Chapter 1), and the diseases can be classified according to which component is deficient. Table 12.1 shows that B cell deficiencies

Table 12.1 Proportion of different types of immune deficiencies

Type of defect	%
B cell deficiency	50
T cell deficiency	35
Phagocytic cell deficiency	18
Complement deficiency	2

comprise the biggest group, followed by deficiencies in T cells. Deficiencies in the complement system are rare.

Diagnosis

Prompt diagnosis of primary immunodeficiency diseases is important as this can lead to life-saving treatment or at least a significant improvement in the patient's quality of life.

Children with normal immune systems can have an average of six to eight respiratory tract infections a year for the first ten years of life and up to six episodes of otitis (ear infections) and two episodes of gastro-enteritis per year for the first two or three years. In some cases, where infants are in day care or have older brothers or sisters at school, incidents of these type of infections may be greater. However, healthy children deal with these infections with no serious problems at all.

In contrast, children with reduced immune systems have more severe infections, which last longer and recur more frequently. Often their infections do not respond to therapies that are commonly used to treat these conditions. Children with immune deficiencies often do not thrive and do not attain normal weight, height and development skills expected for their age. However, some children with immune deficiencies appear to be healthy, and infections are successfully treated with antibiotics. In the early weeks of life, up to three to six months, a child will still have protection from antibodies acquired from the mother before birth. Onset of illness at around six months of age, when maternal antibodies have disappeared, suggests a congenital antibody deficiency. Chronic skin rashes develop in many immunodeficient children within the first year of life. Some primary immune deficiencies occur in infants with other congenital disorders, such as developmental anomalies of the face, skeleton, heart or intestine and disorders of pigmentation and hair.

The nature of the pathogens causing infections can not only suggest that a deficiency in the immune system is present but can also give an indication of its nature.

Infections with gram-positive organisms (pneumococci, streptococci) are common in patients with deficiencies in antibodies (B cells). These infections manifest themselves primarily as recurrent respiratory infections such as pneumonia and are often accompanied by bacterial septicaemia. Patients lacking antibodies are also particularly susceptible to invasive disease with enteroviruses, leading to chronic viral meningitis and to severe and chronic symptoms from gastro-intestinal disease such as giardiasis.

T cells are essential for controlling viral and fungal diseases, so individuals with a defect in this component of the immune system are prone to viral and fungal infections such as thrush. T cells are also important in a helper function to B cells in order to mount an effective antibody response. Thus, individuals with a defect in the T cell component may suffer from immune deficiency diseases caused by both defective T and B cell components and are susceptible to bacterial, chronic and invasive viral and fungal infections.

Patients with deficiencies in the complement component of the immune system have increased susceptibility to conditions such as septic arthritis, meningitis and overwhelming sepsis with *Neisseria meningitidis* and *Neisseria gonorrhoeae.*

Phagocytic diseases include disorders in which the primary defect is one of cell movement (chemotaxis) and others in which it is one of microbicidal activity. Recurrent staphylococcal infections are common in phagocytic deficiencies.

Treatment

Prevention of primary immunodeficiency diseases is limited to genetic counselling for those for which the genetic inheritance pattern is known. Prenatal diagnosis is also possible for some of these disorders and sex determination can be used to exclude X-linked disorders.

Patients with immunodeficiency require an enormous amount of care to maintain optimal health, particularly in managing infections and in preventing emotional problems related to their condition. Substantial costs may also be involved in caring for these individuals. Unnecessary exposure to infection should be avoided. Killed vaccines should be given regularly if there is evidence of some antibody function.

In immunodeficient patients administration of antibiotics is a life-saving treatment. Since these patients often succumb rapidly to infection, antibiotics are given at the first sign of an infection, such as a raised temperature. When the infection does not respond to the initial antibiotic, cultures of the organism are made so that a more appropriate one can be given. Antibiotics given continuously as prophylaxis are sometimes administered, particularly when there is a risk of a sudden overwhelming infection, e.g. Wiskott-Aldrich syndrome. This continuous prophylactic use of antibiotics may also be used when infections keep recurring or there is a high risk for a specific type.

Patients with T or B cell deficiencies should not be given live vaccines, e.g. polio virus, measles, mumps, rubella or BCG, because of the risk of vaccine-induced illness.

Immunoglobulin is an effective replacement therapy in most forms of antibody deficiency. The immunoglobulin consists largely of IgG with trace elements of IgM and IgA. This treatment can be administered either by intravenous or intramuscular injection. It is usually given at monthly intervals but may be more frequent or in stronger concentrations if necessary, e.g. in patients with chronic lung disease.

Plasma has been used instead of immunoglobulin but because of the risk of disease transmission it is not often used. However, in patients who are particularly sensitive to IgA in immunoglobulin, IgA-deficient plasma has been used successfully. Plasma contains many factors in addition to immunoglobulins and is particularly useful in patients with complement deficiencies, protein-losing intestinal conditions and cases of diarrhoea which are difficult to resolve.

Bone marrow transplantation can offer a complete correction of immunodeficiency. In severe combined immunodeficiency and its variants, bone marrow transplantation from an appropriate donor has restored immunity in more than a hundred cases. When using this form of treatment in patients with intact or partial cellular immunodeficiency (e.g. Wiskott-Aldrich syndrome), immunosuppression therapy must be given prior to transplantation to ensure that the graft is not rejected. The ideal donor candidate for this type of transplant is a matched brother or sister. When such a donor is not available, a half-matched bone marrow transplant from a donor parent can be used. However, in this case, mature T lymphocytes, which will cause a graft-versus-host disease (a disease in which donor T cells react against antigens in the immunologically depressed recipient), must be removed from the donor marrow before it is transplanted.

Some of the primary immunodeficiencies are described below.

Bruton's agammaglobulinaemia

Immunodeficiency diseases were first recognised in the early 1950s, and the first disease thought to be caused by a specific defect in the immune system was reported by Dr Ogden Bruton in 1952.

This condition was first recognised in an eight-year-old boy who suffered from repeated bouts of bacterial infection from the age of four onwards. The infection was accompanied by fever, vomiting, joint pain and a variety of other symptoms. The child was treated with penicillin and sulpha drugs, and although this treatment seemed to work initially, the infection returned a short time afterwards with the same symptoms. It was then discovered that the child had no gamma globulin, IgG antibodies. Following treatment with pooled gamma globulin (gamma globulin produced from large pools of donor blood), he was protected from infection for about six years before it began to wear off. Children with this condition have normal immunity to almost all viruses.

This same treatment of antibiotics to clear up ongoing infection followed by pooled human gamma globulin for prophylaxis is used today to treat patients with this condition.

Only young boys are affected by Bruton's agammaglobulinaemia because the gene causing the condition is located on the X-chromosome, also known as a sex chromosome. The condition is described as being X-linked. Girls inherit two X-chromosomes, one from each parent, and so would have to have two defective genes for the condition to manifest itself – which is extremely unlikely.

Combined immunodeficiency

This is a group of disorders that are characterised by a congenital and often hereditary absence of both T cells and B cells, and patients with this condition are susceptible to infection by all microbes. For practical purposes these individuals are identical to patients with Aids.

Onset of these conditions usually occurs within the first three months of life, usually with infections of candidiasis (thrush), pneumonia and diarrhoea. If the condition is left untreated death occurs, usually before the age of two.

In severe combined immunodeficiency (SCID), infections are much more severe as macrophage development is also depressed. Symptoms usually start in infancy, with a failure to thrive, diarrhoea caused by parasitic or viral infection, pneumonia and candidiasis (thrush). Immunisation with live vaccines, e.g. polio, can lead to a fatal infection.

A bone marrow transplant is the recommended treatment, although immunoglobulins and antibiotics can help but do not provide a cure.

DiGeorge syndrome (congenital thymic aplasia)

This syndrome was first described in 1965 and is the result of a failure of the T cell function to develop. Antibody levels are normal. As its name suggests, this is a congenital condition caused by a malformation in the third and fourth pharyngeal pouches in the developing foetus at about four to six weeks of gestation. The thymus and parathyroid are derived primarily from the third and to a lesser extent from the fourth pouch. The parathyroid gland is responsible for regulating blood calcium levels. Patients lacking this gland often suffer convulsions, caused by hypocalcemia, and tetany in infancy – usually within 24 to 48 hours of life. Occurrence of these symptoms at birth is an early indication that T cells are deficient. Several other developmental defects are associated with the syndrome, including cleft palate, nasal clefts, low-set ears and malformations in the major blood vessels and the heart. Severely affected infants often die early from associated cardiac abnormalities. At one time it was thought that this syndrome was an acquired condition caused by a failure of normal embryonic development and not hereditary as there was no familial tendency and both sexes were equally affected. More recently, however, it has been recognised that many cases are associated with structural defects in chromosome 22.

Children with this syndrome have no thymus gland or at most just a little thymus tissue. They are particularly susceptible to viral, bacterial and fungal diseases and have a tendency to develop life-threatening chronic cytomegalovirus and varicella infections. Less severely affected children usually have a few circulating T cells and such infants may remain healthy, with their circulating T cells gradually increasing throughout childhood.

Bone marrow transplantation has been successful in treating this syndrome. In addition, some success has been achieved using foetal thymic transplants in patients with severe conditions.

Wiskott-Aldrich syndrome (WAS)

This disorder, found in male infants, results from a combined deficiency in both T and B cells. There is usually also a mild antibody deficiency with low levels of serum IgM. The first manifestation of the syndrome is bloody diarrhoea, followed by the development of recurrent respiratory infections. Allergic eczema is common, and patients often have high levels of IgE. The combined deficiency in both T and B cell function means that patients are particularly susceptible to viral and fungal infections and some bacterial ones. Malignancy, especially lymphoma, is common in survivors who live beyond ten years old. Patients with this disorder have reduced numbers of platelets, which are also small in size. Removal of the spleen, which is involved in platelet destruction, is often recommended. Other treatments include continuous antibiotics, immune globulins and bone marrow transplantation.

Secondary immunodeficiencies

Malignancies of the lymphatic system, immunosuppressive agents such as those used in the treatment of cancer, transplants and Aids are common causes of severe secondary immunodeficiencies. Nutritional disorders, metabolic disturbances (e.g. uraemia) and trauma have a less severe affect on the immune system. Although in many cases the primary disease usually overshadows the immunodeficiency, appropriate treatment of the latter can improve the quality of life for the patient. A classification of the secondary immunodeficiency diseases is shown in Table 12.2.

As in the primary immunodeficiencies, the type of infection can indicate the nature of the defect in the immune system. Recurrent episodes of pneumonia and bronchitis suggest antibody deficiency, whereas varicella-zoster (shingles) and herpes simplex reactivation, oral thrush and rapid growth of skin warts often indicate a defect in cellular immunity. Some of the more important causes of secondary immunodeficiencies are discussed below.

Cancers

Various cancers, particularly those associated with the lymphatic system, e.g. Hodgkin's disease and lymphoma, can cause immunodeficiency. This may be either a deficiency in antibodies or in T cells. The deficiency is often made worse by the use of cytotoxic drugs that are

Table 12.2: Classification of secondary immunodeficiencies

Premature or newborn infants
Immunodeficiency because of immature immune system

Hereditary and metabolic diseases
Chromosome abnormalities (e.g. Down's syndrome)
Uraemia
Diabetes mellitus
Malnutrition
Vitamin and mineral deficiencies
Protein-losing enteropathies
Nephrotic syndrome
Sickle cell disease

Immunosuppressive agents
Radiation
Immunosuppressive drugs
Corticosteroids
Anti-lymphocyte or anti-thymocyte globulin
Anti-T-cell monoclonal antibodies

Infectious diseases
Congenital rubella
Viral infections e.g. measles, varicella, HIV
Acute bacterial disease
Severe mycobacterial or fungal disease

Haematologic diseases
Hodgkin's disease and lymphoma
Leukaemia
Myeloma
Agranulocytosis and aplastic anaemia

Surgery and trauma
Burns
Splenectomy
Anaesthesia

Miscellaneous
Chronic active hepatitis
Alcoholic cirrhosis
Ageing
Graft-versus-host disease

taken to treat the malignancy. Patients suffering from chronic lymphatic leukaemia have very low levels of gamma globulins and are prone to recurrent infections of the upper and lower respiratory tract. The cause of the deficiency in this antibody is not well understood, but patients benefit from regular replacement of immunoglobulins.

Myeloma, cancer of the bone marrow, is associated with a severe antibody deficiency. Patients with this condition are particularly susceptible to infections of pneumococcal pneumonia and septicaemia. Nowadays, myeloma can be treated with powerful cytotoxic drugs, which can result in prolonged remissions from the disease. Treatment with immunoglobulin can therefore be of benefit to these patients and can greatly improve their quality of life.

Drugs

Many steroid and cytotoxic drugs can seriously depress the immune system. They can have a profound effect on immunity mediated by antibodies. Hence patients on corticosteroids often suffer severe varicella infections (shingles) while patients taking cytotoxic drugs risk infection with cytomegalovirus, which, in the most severe cases, can lead to hepatitis and pneumonitis.

The effects of immunodeficiency caused by drugs is usually reversible although it may take up to two years for antibody production to recover.

Viruses

Human immunodeficiency virus (HIV) is the most well-known immunosuppressive virus. HIV affects the T cells and leads to secondary immunodeficiency syndrome or acquired immunodeficiency syndrome (Aids). Patients with this syndrome become increasingly susceptible to a range of opportunistic infections and tumours. These include herpes and salmonella infections, pneumonia, meningitis, Kaposi's sarcoma and non-Hodgkin's lymphoma.

A number of other viruses may also cause moderate immunosuppression during active infection, the best known of these being measles and cytomegalovirus. These depress cellular immunity. Foetal infection with the rubella virus may, in rare cases, lead to a permanent depression of IgG and IgA antibody production.

Nutritional immunodeficiency

Worldwide, immunodeficiency resulting from poor nutrition is the most common cause and contributes to the high infant death rate in the Third World. Protein-calorie malnutrition and deficiency of vitamins and trace elements, particularly vitamin A, zinc and selenium, can lead to a reduction of T lymphocyte function as well as poor antibody production. Vitamin A supplements have been shown to reduce childhood mortality from infection in some populations.

Severe trauma and burns

In these conditions both antibody and lymphocyte function can be affected. The deficiency of antibodies is of limited importance where broad-spectrum antibiotics are in routine use. The longer a critical illness persists, the more likely it is that the reduction of T lymphocytes becomes clinically important. Patients who are critically ill for a prolonged period often die from cytomegalovirus or fungal infections. Immunosuppression is often pronounced in young children who have suffered severe burns and antibody production may be severely reduced.

Ageing

A degree of immunodeficiency usually occurs as a consequence of increasing age. The thymus, which is important in the production of T cells, reaches a peak in size in puberty and after that begins to shrink steadily. This results in the decline in the number and activity of T lymphocytes and also a reduction in the number of B cells.

13

Transplantation and the Immune System

Transplantation can be defined as the transfer of living tissues or cells from a donor to a recipient with the intention of maintaining vital functions. So, for example, a transplanted heart is expected to carry out the functions once performed by the heart that had to be removed.

The knowledge, skills, techniques and understanding of organ transplants has developed tremendously over the last 30 years since the first kidneys were transplanted in the 1950s and the first heart in 1967. Transplantation of organs is now common practice, and the rate of success that can be achieved would have seemed unlikely only ten years ago. There has been an enormous expansion in the role of transplant surgery in treating patients whose organs, e.g. the kidneys, have failed completely. This is known as *end-stage organ failure*. Patients are often faced with a choice of renal dialysis for the rest of their lives or a transplant. In the case of other body organs, machines may not be available to take over their roles, so a transplant may be the only hope of survival. Transplantation is now performed in people of all ages, from babies only a few days old to people in their seventies.

Survival rates in patients receiving all types of transplants have improved over the last 20 years. Of the patients receiving kidney and heart transplants, over 80 per cent have an organ that is still in place and functioning well a year after the procedure is carried out. Success for liver transplants has more than doubled in the last ten years, from a 30 per cent survival rate in 1980 to a 75 per cent survival rate in 1990.

The expansion of transplant surgery and the improved survival rates are the result of a number of factors. These include improved surgical techniques, better patient selection, earlier transplantation, a more selective use of immunosuppressive drugs, improved matching of donor and recipient tissue, an earlier and more accurate detection of rejection and a better understanding of the immune mechanisms involved.

The initial attempts at transplant surgery over 30 years ago were carried out in the face of considerable ignorance about the nature of the immune response. Today, despite the technical feasibility of transplanting any tissue, mainly because of improved surgical techniques, the value of such transplants is still limited. One of the main obstacles is the rejection reaction, which can destroy the tissue soon after transplantation. Understanding of the rejection mechanism is now a rapidly expanding area of knowledge. As understanding of the immune mechanism involved in transplant rejection increases, better methods of monitoring and controlling the process with more specific immunosuppressive drugs can be developed.

Transplants are categorised by site and the genetic relationship between donor and recipient. These are outlined in Table 13.1 below.

Table 13.1: Categories of transplants

autograft (**autogeneic graft**)	transfer of self tissue from one location to another, e.g. one graft to stabilise a fracture, a skin graft to treat severe burns.
isograft (**syngeneic graft**)	a graft between identical twins
allograft (**allogeneic** or **homograft**)	a graft between genetically dissimilar members of the same species
xenograft (**xenogeneic** or **heterograft**)	transplant between members of different species

The majority of transplants are allografts, i.e. grafts from one person to another. The donor may be a living relative or a person who has recently died. Living donors are accepted only in the case of kidney or bone marrow transplants. However, there have been a number of experimental transplants using small parts of the liver and pancreas donated by living relatives of the recipient.

The number of people waiting for transplants far outweighs the quantity of suitable organs that are available, either from living relatives or from dead donors.

The immunology of transplantation

The rejection of transplanted organs is a normal function of a properly working immune system, which, in the majority of cases, acts to protect the body against disease-causing organisms. The main features of the immune system have been described earlier in this book (Chapter 1), and it is not surprising to find that the mechanisms involved in the rejection of a transplant are broadly similar to those active in dealing with any 'foreign body'. In addition to these mechanisms, however, there are a number of special features implicated in the rejection of a transplant. These features can be considered under two main headings. First, the steps involved in implementing the response (sensitisation) and, second, the mechanisms involved in destroying the transplant.

Major histocompatibility antigens

In the rejection of a transplant, it is the antigens present on the cell membrane of the tissue that are immediately

recognised as 'foreign'. More precisely, it is the glyco-
proteins on the cell membrane that are the antigens.
These antigens are referred to as *histocompatibility antigens* or *transplantation antigens*, and it is these antigens that determine the outcome of transplants between
members of the same species. Rejection of a transplant
is effected through both the cellular components of the
immune system and antibodies reacting against the cell
membrane antigens.

These antigens can be divided into *major* and *minor
histocompatibility antigens*. The major histocompatibility antigens are under the genetic control of one system
called the *major histocompatibility complex* (*MHC*),
and the minor histocompatibility antigens are under the
control of a number of systems – at least 40 but possibly
as many as several hundred. It is the incompatibility of
the MHC between the donor and the recipient that is
thought to lead to the immune response against the
transplant and its ultimate destruction. The minor histocompatibility antigens appear to play little part in the
rejection process except in cases where there is no incompatibility between the MHC but a number of minor
differences exist between the minor histocompatibility
antigens. In these cases the transplant can also be rejected. Little is known about the minor histocompatibility
systems in human beings, but evidence for their exist-
ence comes from the observation that rejection of kidney and bone marrow transplants between identical
twins with identical MHC has occurred.

In humans, the MHC is referred to as *human leucocyte group A (HLA)* antigens. HLA, together with the major blood group (ABO) antigens are the chief transplantation antigens known at present.

Rejection of transplants

Rejection of transplanted organs or tissues may occur almost immediately (*hyperacute rejection*) or over longer time periods (*acute rejection* and *late graft rejection*). Various mechanisms are employed in each type.

The immune response in the rejection of transplants is mediated by both T cells and antibody. T helper cells are critical in the immune response in patients who are not previously sensitised, while T cytotoxic cells have a role but are not essential. In patients who have been sensitised, the T cytotoxic cells are the prime effectors of the response. Other cells, such as macrophages, have a secondary role, and antibodies also play a part in acute and late graft rejection.

Acute rejection

Acute rejection is a delayed hypersensitivity Type II response (*see* Chapter 1) which causes destruction of the graft within days or months after transplantation. At first the transplant process seems to be going well and the organs or tissues begin to function as expected. However, within a few days they begin to lose these functions and, in the case of skin grafts, the skin becomes purplish and then black. By the end of the eleventh to seventeenth day, the graft has been rejected. This type of rejection is characterised by infiltration of the allograft by several immune system cell types, including macrophages, lymphocytes and other plasma cells. Varying degrees of haemorrhage and swelling occur, although the blood vessels remain generally intact. Cell-mediated rejection may be reversed in many cases by increasing immunosuppressive therapy. Where the reversal of the rejection process is successful, examination of the graft shows that the damaged parts heal with some scarring and the remainder appears normal. Such transplants often survive for prolonged periods, even though immunosuppressive therapy is reduced to very low levels. This so-called 'graft adaptation' is thought to be the result of the development of donor-specific suppression of the recipient's immune response.

Late graft deterioration

Deterioration of the graft some time after transplantation occurs occasionally in patients who are undergoing immunosuppressive therapy. This type of rejection often proceeds insidiously despite increased drug therapy. It is thought to be the result of antibody-mediated damage. The membranes lining the blood vessels are primarily involved, with the vessels eventually becoming blocked and so cutting off the blood supply to the graft, leading to its ultimate destruction.

Hyperacute rejection

Hyperacute rejection usually occurs in individuals who have been presensitised to HLA antigens present in the graft. Presensitisation may be because of pregnancy, blood transfusion or a previous transplant. The role of antibodies to the transplantation antigens in the rejection of the graft is obvious in these cases. Destruction of the graft occurs within hours or even minutes of the transplant being connected to the host blood system.

This antibody-mediated rejection involves components of the complement system, phagocytes and macrophages. These act so quickly that the graft never has an opportunity to take. The graft may become engorged with blood, which may coagulate within the donor organ. This can occur so rapidly that the transplanted organ has to be removed, literally within minutes. The death of the graft cannot be reversed by any known immunosuppressive techniques. Liver grafts seem to be less susceptible to this form of antibody-mediated hyperacute rejection. Antibody-mediated rejection is also probably important in delayed graft destruction but its exact role is not yet well understood.

A similar rejection, mediated by antibodies, usually occurs if a transplant is carried out between donors and recipients whose blood groups do not match. This is similar to the reaction that occurs in blood transfusions as the antigens involved are present on all cells of the body. So, for example, if cells bearing A type antigens are transferred to a blood group O or B individual, the anti-A haemagglutinin combines with the tissue to initiate typical destruction. It is therefore important, when evaluating the suitability of a transplant, that there must be compatibility between the blood groups of the recipient and donor.

Suitability for transplant

To determine whether tissues are suitable for transplanting into a specific individual, the HLA antigens present in both the donor and recipient are investigated. Only those tissues that share common HLA antigens are considered suitable for use. The principal target of the immune response in a vascularised transplant such as a kidney is the endothelium, which contains both Class I and Class II antigens.

Graft versus host rejection

The graft versus host rejection (GVHR) develops when immunocompetent tissues (i.e. tissues that can mount an immune response) are transferred to an immuno-handicapped host. This may happen naturally when maternal lymphoid tissue is transferred to the foetus during pregnancy. The rejected tissue does not always die.

Mild reversible GVHR is more frequent when the donor and host share a good degree of histocompatibility but are not identical. This type of rejection was observed when surgeons transplanted bone marrow and thymus tissue to children with proven immunodeficiencies. There was some mild rejection of the tissue, but the tissue survived and repopulated the host with immunocompetent cells.

Privileged sites and privileged tissues

These are certain sites within the body in which allografted tissue does not evoke an immune response and grafts can survive for prolonged periods or even indefinitely. The best known of these 'privileged sites' in humans is the cornea. When corneas are transplanted, they can restore vision. and the success of this technique has led to it becoming a standard procedure, with about 3500 being performed each year in Britain. The cornea contains no vascularised tissue and is therefore protected from the lymphatic system and immune system components.

As well as privileged sites, there are also 'privileged tissues', which are less susceptible to rejection. Tissues in this category include bone cartilage, heart valves, sections of the aorta and other major blood vessels, and tendons. Bone and cartilage can be preserved indefinitely in a lyophilised state or frozen, and can be rehydrated or thawed and immediately ready for use.

The foetus is an example of a privileged tissue *par excellence*. It was thought that the uterus was a privileged site, but when other tissues are transplanted to this organ they are rejected, and so it appears that the pregnant uterus has some special characteristics. A layer of tissue, the prohoblast layer, physically separates the uterine wall from the tissues of the foetus. Each cell in this layer of tissue surrounds itself with a mucoprotein. When the mother and foetus are only distantly related antigenically, this layer of mucoprotein is substantial. When the mother and foetus are antigenically close, little mucoprotein is found. The trophoblastic layer therefore appears to protect the developing foetus from the mother's immune system.

Immunosuppression

Although nowadays transplant donors and recipients are matched as far as possible to decrease the possibility of rejection, some form of immunosuppressive therapy is nearly always used. In the 1950s, when the first kidney transplants were performed, the majority of them were rejected. By the 1960s there was evidence that certain drugs such as 6–mercaptopurine and its derivative, azathioprine, prolonged kidney allografts in animals. Since then virtually all human transplant patients have received some sort of immunosuppression therapy, and this is primarily responsible for the present success of transplant surgery. Intensive immunosuppression is usually required only during the first few weeks after a transplant or during a rejection crisis. After that, the graft often seems to become accommodated and only small doses of immunosuppressive drugs are required. Today, the goal of medication is to create a situation in which the transplant is tolerated by the recipient without the need for a lifetime of drug taking.

Immunosuppression therapy depresses the action of the immune system. The early drugs used in this type of therapy suppressed all aspects of the immune system, leaving patients more liable to suffer from infections of all sorts. Infection then became the leading cause of death among transplant patients. By the late 1960s, a combination of corticosteroids and azathioprine had been shown to be an effective regime for increasing the chance of a successful organ transplant. Besides the side effects of skin rashes, diarrhoea, nausea and vomiting, transplant patients taking azathioprine were also at an increased risk of developing various cancers, including tumours of the skin, lymphomas and occasionally leukaemias. The immune system is involved in tracking down and eliminating cancer-causing cells. In patients undergoing treatment to suppress the system, these potential cancer-causing cells find the compromised host ideal for their proliferation.

In 1972, a new drug, cyclosporin A, was discovered. This drug was isolated from a fungus growing in the soil in Norway. It is a potent immunosuppressant and has relatively low toxic side effects. It has a variety of effects on the immune system; perhaps most importantly, it can suppress the actions of the T cells and so can act to inhibit the rejection of a transplanted organ. Cyclosporin A acts only on the T cells involved in the immune response to the graft, and if it is given before these encounter the transplant, it can prevent them from becoming activated. Cyclosporin A does not affect other T cells not involved in the rejection of the transplant, leaving them alive and healthy to participate in other immune responses as required. It also had fewer side effects than other drugs that were in current usage at that time.

Clinical trials of cyclosporin A were started in 1983. Prior to this time, over 50 per cent of kidney transplants failed. After the introduction of Cyclosporin A, the failure rate for this type of transplant fell to only 15 per cent. Similarly, the success rate for heart transplants doubled after the introduction of cyclosporin, and the average hospitalisation for this type of procedure was reduced from 70 to 40 days. The side effects of cyclosporin A include nausea and excessive hair growth. The major limitation on the use of this drug is its toxicity, particularly in relation to the kidneys.

Developments in immunotherapy

Many new immunosuppressive drugs are undergoing extensive clinical trials. None of these drugs will be perfect, but they control different forms of rejection and act more specifically on different parts of the immune system. One of these drugs, known as FK506, which is also derived from a soil fungus, works in the same way as cyclosporin A by suppressing T cells. It is as effective as cyclosporin A but less toxic. Another drug undergoing trials, Rapamycin, which was discovered in a soil microbe, acts in a different way to block T cells. It is likely that use of various combinations of these newer drugs will be more effective, less toxic and more specific than the ones that are used currently.

Other developments in transplant techniques include the transfer of stem cells (primitive cells that give rise to various blood cells, including lymphocytes) from umbilical cord blood of newly born infants to patients whose bone marrow activity has been destroyed as a result of radiation and chemotherapy, as in the treatment of leukaemia. Stem cells from the umbilical cord stand less chance of being rejected because they have a poorly developed immune response, and in this respect they are more suitable for transplants than bone marrow. So far in Britain, this technique has been used to treat children with bone marrow deficiencies, using stem cells from their newly born brothers or sisters. Cord blood can be stored for long periods, and banks are being set up in Britain to store this for possible use with other patients.

The future of transplantation

Although in the past the rejection of transplants has been the biggest barrier to success, the great strides forward that have been made in the last 15 years means that this will be less of a problem in the future. Other factors are likely to become more important in the development of transplant surgery. The most prominent of these is the availability of organs for transplant. As the success of transplant surgery has increased, so has the demand for more organs. With the exception of bone marrow and some kidney transplants from living close relatives, organs for transplant purposes depend on someone else's death.

With the advent of seat-belt legislation and improved medical and surgical techniques, the availability of organs for donation has decreased. Currently there are some 6000 people in Britain waiting for transplants, many of whom will die before they receive such an operation. Research is being carried out to investigate the use of animal organs for human transplants. This, of course, raises many ethical questions concerning the use of animals, not to mention the possibility of transferring diseases to humans who receive such transplants. This latter problem has been highlighted recently in the case of corneas that were transplanted from a woman to three donors. It was later found that the donor was infected with Creutzfeldt-Jakob disease, leaving the recipients at possible risk of contracting the disease via their transplants.

Glossary

acute the term used to describe a short-lived disease or condition that starts rapidly with severe symptoms.

adrenaline (epinephrine) a natural hormone produced by the adrenal glands during exercise or when a person is under stress or frightened. Adrenaline acts on the blood vessels to maintain normal blood pressure and circulation. It can be given by injection or inhaler to treat the symptoms of severe allergic reactions such as anaphylaxis or asthma.

allergen any substance, usually a protein, that causes an allergic reaction. Once an allergy has developed, even small amounts of the substance can cause an allergic response.

allergy an abnormal or inappropriate reaction of the immune system to a previously encountered substance (an allergen), which would normally be harmless.

antibody *or* **immunoglobulin** a protein produced by the immune system in response to the presence of a foreign substance (antigen). Antibodies circulate in the blood and help in the fight against infection. The antibody immunoglobulin E (IgE) is involved in triggering allergic reactions, and high levels of IgE are found in atopic individuals.

antigen an invading substance that provokes an immune response.

atopy an hereditary tendency to develop Type I allergic reactions, such as asthma, hay fever and eczema.

autoimmune the term used to describe a disordered response of the immune system directed against a constituent of the individual's own body.

chronic a disorder or condition that is long lasting. It may be mild or severe and will often involve some long-term or permanent change in the body.

dander tiny particles of animal skin and the scales from animal hair or fur which can act as an allergen.

degranulation release of chemical mediators of allergy such as histamine, prostaglandins and leukotrienes from mast cells. Degranulation occurs when an allergen bridges across adjacent IgE molecules.

desensitisation *or* **immunotherapy** a treatment for allergy in which injections of gradually increasing amounts of allergen are given over a period of several months in an attempt to reduce or eliminate symptoms by building up the immune system's tolerance to the substance.

eosinophil a white blood cell that is present at the site of an allergic reaction, in parasitic worm infestation and in reactions to certain drugs.

epinephrine *see* **adrenaline**.

histamine one of the main constituents of the granules in mast cells and an active mediator in allergic reactions, particularly potent in tightening muscles in the airways and in inflammation as well as in other symptoms of allergy.

hypersensitive a term meaning allergic.

immunodeficiency a general term implying that the immune system is in some way defective. This may be the result of an inherited or acquired defect, as may occur following exposure to HIV.

immunoglobulins a family of proteins to which antibodies belong. *See* **antibody**.

immunotherapy *see* **desensitisation**.

immunosuppressive drugs drugs that are capable of suppressing the immune response.

leukotriene one of the chemical mediators of allergy.

lymphocyte a type of white blood cell important in immunity and allergy, there are two major types – T lymphocytes and B lymphocytes.

mast cell a type of cell found in body tissues that contains packets of chemicals which, when released, cause the symptoms of allergy.

phagocyte a cell of the immune system that responds to contact with a foreign object, such as a bacterium, by surrounding, engulfing and digesting it.

prostaglandins a group of hormones that are found throughout tissues and body fluids and involved in many body functions. They are important in the constriction of smooth muscle in allergic reactions. They also commonly stimulate pain nerve endings, and many analgesic drugs act by preventing the release of prostaglandins from injured tissue.

sensitise to expose to an allergen for the first time, which will provoke a response in the immune system upon subsequent encounters.

T cell *or* **T lymphocyte** a type of white blood cell that is responsible for cell-mediated immunity, i.e. they attack foreign agents such as viruses directly. Some T cells act as 'helper' cells and provide assistance to B lymphocytes in producing antibodies. Absence of helper T cells results in the inability of the immune system to protect the body against infection, as in Aids.

topical a term used to describe the way in which a drug is applied directly to the affected part.